T0304855

Hour
of
the
Heart

IRVIN D. YALOM
AND BENJAMIN YALOM

Hour
of
the
Heart

PIATKUS

First published in United States of America in 2024 by Harper, an imprint of
HarperCollins Publishers

First published in Great Britain in 2024 by Piatkus

1 3 5 7 9 10 8 6 4 2

A CIP catalogue record for this book
is available from the British Library.

ISBN: 978-0-34943-671-5 (Hardback)
ISBN: 978-0-34943-672-2 (Trade paperback)

Printed and bound in Great Britain by Clays Ltd, Elcograf S.p.A.

Papers used by Piatkus are from well-managed forests and other responsible sources.

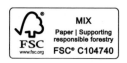

Piatkus
An imprint of
Little, Brown Book Group
Carmelite House
50 Victoria Embankment
London EC4Y 0DZ

The authorised representative
in the EEA is
Hachette Ireland
8 Castlecourt Centre, Dublin 15,
D15 XTP3, Ireland
(email: info@hbgi.ie)

An Hachette UK Company
www.hachette.co.uk

www.littlebrown.co.uk

For my children, Eve, Reid, Victor, and Ben; their children; and their children's children.

—IRVIN D. YALOM

For Anisa, who makes my heart trill and quiver every day.

—BENJAMIN YALOM

Contents

Introduction

I once had the audacious idea to compile my most important insights about how to do psychotherapy into what became a useful book called *The Gift of Therapy*. In its introduction I wrote that, at the ripe age of seventy, two things were happening for me. First, my patients had begun to worry how long I would be around to help them. Would I go on vacation and never return? Might they soon be visiting my grave? Second, given my seemingly imminent demise, I found myself wanting to pass on what I had learned in my four decades as a psychotherapist, and to do so as quickly as possible.

These fears have proved just the slightest bit premature and, more than twenty years later, I am still contemplating how to best help patients and therapists alike. Now, as I sneak up on age ninety-three, perhaps concerns such as my death and the need to pass on hard-earned lessons truly are pressing. I can't be sure. Check back with me in another twenty years or so!

One thing that has been consistent in my now *six* decades as a therapist is that the longing for human connection is a main force that drives those seeking help. People crave closer, better relationships. Key to developing these rich relationships are the ability, and the willingness, to open up, to share intimate space with others. This may sound easy enough, and yet the vast majority of patients I've encountered have difficulties doing so. Intimacy requires vulnerability: you can't expect your friend, relative, or partner to be open to you unless you are willing to be open to them. And such vulnerability, almost by definition, does not feel safe. Many of us—*most of us*—have had experiences in which emotional vulnerability has gone awry. It felt dreadful, and we quickly developed defenses, foremost among them learning not to allow ourselves to open up again. But, alas, if we never allow ourselves to open up, we never get the connection we crave.

For those familiar with my work in existential psycho-therapy, this emphasis on interpersonal connection may seem incongruous. In fact, rereading the introduction to *The Gift of Therapy*, I note that I discussed the two as "parallel but separate interests." Existential psychotherapy focuses on patients' inner conflicts that arise from confronting the givens of human existence—death, isolation, meaning in life, and freedom. I noted that this existential lens (for it is not a dis-crete, complete approach to therapy) informed my work with individuals. With interpersonal therapy, on the other hand, I assume that patients struggle because they are unable to develop, nurture, and maintain close relationships with others. I located this primarily in my work with therapy groups, where I focused on the exchanges, impulses, and emotions that arose from the members' responses to one another.

I feel now that these two sets of concerns may not be so dis-tinct after all. One of the great drivers of existential anxiety is our condition of being alone in the universe, such that we can never completely share our experience with another. This ultimate isolation can be terrifying, and certainly plays a role in the theology of most religions, which offer solace by assuring us we are part of a greater whole. For many of us, whether we are religious or not, deep connection with other people is the best salve for that isolation and the anxieties that come with it. In this sense, when I say that most people come to therapy looking for help with interpersonal problems, this feels quite related to existential concerns.

Likewise, while the stories that make up this book are all about working one on one with individual patients, the approach I employ is explicitly interpersonal, mining the here and now of the emotional space between the two of us and using what we learn from this to help the patient get better at relating with others. So, again, the existential and the interpersonal are not so separate.

This need for connection to ease the existential concerns has certainly been true for me, brought into sharp focus after my wife of sixty-five years, Marilyn, died in 2019. COVID appeared just months later, and I spent much of the following three years, the time frame of this book, in heavy isolation. Add to that the fact that I had entered *serious* old man territory. Nearly all of my friends and colleagues had passed away, or seemed to be doing so as quickly as possible. Living to a ripe old age, while maybe better than the alternative, has its drawbacks.

Existential issues have been much on my mind as I've aged. One major feature of aging has been the decline of my memory. Because examining its deterioration is a major feature of this book, I won't reveal much in this introduction, other than to touch on two critical aspects. First, six years ago I determined that I could no longer remember all the important details of my patients' lives and the therapy work we had done together. I simply could not promise to be the effective therapist I'd been for so long. Rather than take down my shingle immediately, I chose to offer single consultations to those in need. The most compelling of these consultations, and the lessons gleaned from them, are the core of the chapters that follow.

Second, while the stories here are told in my, Irvin Yalom's, voice, the writing is truly a collaboration between myself and my youngest son, Benjamin. We came upon this interesting arrangement out of necessity, as I found myself unable to hold the many encounters described here, and the related therapeutic threads, in my mind at the same time. Fortunately Ben is an excellent writer who has edited my work for many years. The timing could not have been better: after twenty-five years working in the theater and, he says, avoiding being in my professional shadow, this prodigal son decided to join the family business. He was in the middle of his PhD studies in marriage and family therapy when my aspirations for this book slammed up against the reality of my crumbling mind. What has resulted is a rich combination of my experiences and his observations and insightful questions. What luck! It has been a delight to collaborate, to be challenged to clarify and rethink some of my assumptions, and to have him as one of my last students through our work on these pages.

Terminology and a Critical Caveat

Lastly, a few notes of guidance. Two terms used frequently throughout the book are worth clarifying. First, I speak often of *intimacy*. I am not using this term to describe anything sexual or physical, even as that seems to be a common usage in our culture today. Rather I am discussing closeness, affection, familiarity—any slew of words that might indicate a warm, tender opening of people to one another. Therapy, as illustrated in these stories, should be a safe space for experiencing and practicing this intimacy.

Second, I refer to the people who have come to me for consultations as *patients*. This term is a bit problematic. The field of psychotherapy was originated by psychiatrists, who were trained medical doctors, and thus referred quite naturally to their *patients*. In recent decades, however, psychotherapy has become largely the domain of psychologists, marriage and family therapists, social workers, and counselors of various sorts, most of whom use the term *clients*. I am not an enormous fan of either of these words—one seems to imply disease, and the other commerce—nor is there a term closer related to consultation (*consultor?*) that rolls off the tongue without offending the ear. I prefer to think of myself as a *fellow traveler*—one who has, perhaps, a slightly better view of the road we are traveling. Nonetheless, in these stories, I've used *patients*, despite the fact that I was not offering ongoing care, nor intending to take on any medical responsibility.

Finally, this is a collection about single-session encounters with people seeking guidance. From over three hundred such encounters I have selected twenty-two stories that are intended to help teach therapists and those interested in therapy, to pass on specific lessons, or to reveal particular dilemmas. Let me state in the clearest possible of terms that *I am not suggesting that a single session should be seen as an effective model of therapy!* It should be superfluous to put this caveat here, but given that our field has been driven by insurance and pharmacology companies to shorter and increasingly

XVI • Introduction

impoverished versions of what therapy might be, I feel the need to clarify. My hope is not that my experiment will be replicated, but that you, dear readers, can take the lessons passed on here and incorporate them into your own practices in the ways you find most helpful.

HOUR OF THE HEART

CHAPTER I

A Day in the Life of a Very Old Therapist

The day had not started well. I woke at 3:00 a.m. with leg cramps that wouldn't go away. I quietly got out of bed, careful not to disturb my wife, Marilyn, sleeping deeply next to me. To relieve the pain I took a hot shower until it turned lukewarm, then dried myself and returned to bed. The heat had soothed my muscles, and the cramps had subsided somewhat. I tried hard to go back to sleep. But when it comes to sleep, "trying hard" is always doomed to failure. Insomnia has been my kryptonite for decades.

I had been tapering down my use of sleeping pills, reluctantly, as my doctor suspected they were accelerating my memory loss. I tried some breathing exercises. Time after time I inhaled, whispering "calm," and exhaled, whispering "ease," a meditation practice I'd learned years ago. But it was to no avail—the slight calming brought on by the utterance of "ease" soon morphed into anxiety, another old nemesis. I shifted my attention and focused on counting my breaths. A couple of minutes later I realized I had forgotten about counting and my ever-restless mind had wandered elsewhere.

A year earlier Marilyn had been diagnosed with multiple myeloma, an insidious cancer of the blood plasma. She was in the midst of a series of chemotherapy treatments, which had yet to result in any significant improvement. Her warmth and the sound of her breathing were so familiar, my beloved bedmates for many decades. But now something new had joined us, this sinister illness, doing battle within her.

I was pleased to see her resting peacefully that night and gently traced the lines of her face in the dim light. We'd been together, inseparable, since middle school. Now I spent the majority of my days worrying about her and trying to enjoy the time we still had together. Nights I spent worrying about a life without her. How would I pass the time? With whom would I share my thoughts? What loneliness awaited me?

Noticing that my mind had strayed so thoroughly, I gave up the idea of getting back to sleep. I checked the clock and noted, to my surprise, that it was already 6:00 a.m. Somehow, when I wasn't paying attention, I must have nodded off for a couple of hours.

After breakfast, I looked at my schedule. I had only two appointments that day. The first was a termination, the final session with Jerry, a patient whom I'd been seeing for one year. Jerry was a successful lawyer in his forties who had come to therapy seeking answers after his girlfriend of two years had left him, the third in a string of failed relationships.

"I can't see why," he'd said during our first meeting. "I've got a great house, a great job, tons of money. What's not to like? I mean look at me." He'd gestured at the well-tailored, clearly expensive suit he was wearing.

Jerry was not what you'd call warm or reassuring. He was demanding, and often critical. He groused about my fee, suggested I get a better gardener to tend the plants along the walkway to my office, and, once inside, disparaged the artwork on the walls.

He had come to me, he told me repeatedly during our first few meetings, because he'd heard I was the best, and he deserved the best. This was soon accompanied by a look of disappointment in his eyes that I hadn't swiftly cured him of his troubles. Clearly, that look said I wasn't the best after all.

And yet, over time, we'd had success. What had worked? We had two important factors going for us. First, Jerry was highly motivated to make change in his life. Despite his prickly exterior he realized that he was in some way contributing to his relationship problems, and he was eager to put in whatever work was needed to address this. I had to slow him down, let him breathe, and see that part of the problem was the immense demands he placed on himself and on me to magically "fix" him.

"Imagine being your girlfriend for a few minutes," I suggested. "What if you weren't 'the best,' if your garden path weren't expertly tended, if you didn't look perfect on Jerry's arm? Would Jerry love you and support you nonetheless?"

"I doubt it," he said.

"Instead he would criticize you constantly, and you'd end up feeling crappy about yourself and your relationship. And . . . ?" I left the question hanging in the air.

Jerry considered for a moment.

"And you probably wouldn't stick around," he said finally.

This realization, that being demanding and often unkind severely impacted his relationships, clicked for him. He could see the role he was playing and started to change. In the weeks that followed, he set about in earnest to improve. He began to catch himself whenever he was overly critical of me and whenever he complained that others in his life were inadequate. He took more responsibility for the way people, especially potential romantic partners, responded to him. And he set about curbing his sharp tongue. Jerry's fierce drive to change himself was essential to the progress he made, but it was not something I could control.

I *could* influence another factor, however, the powerful relationship he and I developed. From the beginning Jerry had tested me: Why wasn't my taste in art better? Where was my fancy car? Why hadn't I been able to fix him all the way yet? Through all these barbs I'd stayed in there with him. I'd been empathetic and warm, and also willing to push back when it seemed a challenge would do him some good. Gradually he softened up and stopped competing with me. As our relationship grew, his bristles felt less like attacks and more like witty, playful jabs that I could parry or call him out on. Little by little we built a strong connection, a "therapeutic alliance" as we call it in the field.

This alliance, building it and using it, is the most important factor in my therapeutic approach. In what now seem like countless lectures, and numerous writings, I've stated that "it is the relationship that heals." What drives change is not a worksheet that the patient fills out, a brilliant question the therapist poses, or a behavioral change the patient must chart daily. In my approach to therapy the honest connection between the therapist and the patient is the medium through which we discover, learn, change, and heal.

Jerry and I had made excellent progress using that relationship over the course of the year we had together. He became friendlier, and when he occasionally still snapped at me with a disapproving comment, I would point it out. He learned to apologize and then, bit by bit, catch himself before saying something acerbic, and often, quite endearingly, replace such comments with attempts at compliments: "The lemon trees beside the path are looking much better this week" or "You know, that statue of Buddha on your bookshelf is actually more interesting that I thought."

I looked forward to our weekly meetings and would be sad to say goodbye when today's session ended at 11:50. But, for reasons that will become clear, we had agreed upon a one-year time frame at the beginning of his therapy. He had certainly made the most of it, and we were both hopeful that his future relationships, romantic and otherwise, would be richer and more satisfying.

The second session on my schedule that day would be very different. It was with a woman named Susan, whom I planned to see only once. Only once!? How could I do anything resembling effective therapy in a single session? And why would I want to try? To explain, I need to rewind my timeline a bit to provide context.

About five years before this, when I was in my early eighties, I noticed that my memory was starting to fail. I had always been a bit forgetful, misplacing my appointment book, glasses, or car keys with regularity. This was something different. I began to encounter people I recognized, only to have their names elude me. Occasionally I'd stop in the middle of a sentence, stuck searching for a familiar word. And, more and more frequently, I would lose track of the characters in movies Marilyn and I were watching.

As this progressed I began to think that, perhaps, I was no longer able to offer the long-term therapy I had for nearly sixty years. Instead of open-ended therapy that sometimes lasted three or four years, I decided to set a twelve-month time limit, agreed upon in advance, for all new patients. Hence my agreement with Jerry. I approached this new framework with some sense of loss, as it represented a major shift in my work, one derived from necessity, not desire. But soon curiosity, and my wish to continue being helpful, won out.

Ultimately I found this to be an agreeable solution. If I chose my patients carefully, I was almost always able to offer a great deal during our year's work together. With some patients, in fact, there was an increased sense of urgency, and thus motivation, thanks to the time limitation. This had worked well, both for me and for my patients, for the last five years. Then around the time I was eighty-seven, I started to find I was more and more reliant on the summaries I recorded after each session to remember the details of my patients and that, even with these notes in hand, their faces and problems occasionally seemed alien. I was faltering, and I began to question the value of the care I was able to provide. I felt I still had much to offer, but it was clear that I could not, in good conscience, engage in ongoing work with patients, even limited to one year.

And yet, and yet . . . the thought of no longer practicing was dizzying. Sharing with my patients, aiding them through their darkest thoughts, and joining them on journeys of discovery—for the majority of my life this had been my daily work, and my calling. Who would I be, if not a psychotherapist? Truth be told I was angry and deeply frightened. I was not ready to feel this old, this useless. The thought of leaving therapy behind felt like resigning myself to rapid decline, followed soon after by my inevitable death.

I pondered this dilemma. I had to put my patients' needs first, so doing long-term therapy was out. But after so many decades of practice and research, I knew I had developed levels of insight and expertise that were rare, and still potent. Plus I felt the personal need to continue contributing in some way. How could I offer something—enough to be helpful to patients, enough to keep myself engaged in the world—while also not endangering anyone? I came up with an unconventional idea. Perhaps I could meet with people for onetime, one-hour, consultations. During that hour I would offer everything I could—insight, guidance, a warm accepting presence—and then, if appropriate, refer them to a colleague who seemed well attuned to their particular challenges for ongoing treatment.

The idea of such short-course therapy was profoundly foreign to me. I have always seen therapy as a longer-term endeavor—not the endless years of old-school psychoanalysis, but often several years, long enough to help patients search for better understanding of themselves and make meaningful change in their lives. The question of how I might be effective in single sessions could be an interesting experiment, if nothing else.

For some time after coming up with this idea I vacillated between skepticism—was this just a way of forestalling my own decline rather than offering anything truly beneficial to the patients?—and excitement—I knew I had skills honed to an uncommon degree and had been helpful to many, many struggling people, which undoubtedly had some value. I took the time to stare carefully at my own feelings. It was possible my pride would resist accepting this position of lessened importance. And yet I knew that, at some point, I would need to accept my decline and pass the torch fully to the next generations. I honestly did not know what this experiment would yield, which itself was intriguing. Thus I began a new adventure of short therapeutic encounters, and investigation of what might be most helpful in a far briefer time frame for motivating change than I had ever before conceived as effective.

I announced my retirement from ongoing therapy, and my offer of these single-hour consultations—either in person in my Palo Alto office or online—on my Facebook page. Within hours, requests for appointments started to pour in, far more than I'd expected. They came from all over the world, English-speaking countries of course, but also many other places, too—Turkey, Greece, Israel, Germany—as Zoom had collapsed the barrier of space. And they came from people in many stages, and to some extent many walks, of life. This single-session format, I quickly realized, would allow me to work with many people I had never been able to reach otherwise, people for whom ongoing therapy with me was prohibitively expensive. It was clear this would be a very interesting shift from the relatively traditional private practice I'd led from the lovely Spanish-style cottage in our backyard over the previous twenty years, and for decades before that working in the psychiatry department at Stanford University. Would it be effective for the patients? Would it feel satisfying for me? Only time would tell. It would certainly be new, and at my age newness was nothing to scoff at.

This, then, was how I found myself on that particular morning contemplating my first single-session consultation with Susan. I was excited yet concerned. I am not always filled with second-guessing, but after a restless night spent with my darker thoughts about Marilyn's failing body and my own weakening mind, I had my doubts. How much good would I be able to do, really, in these short encounters?

I had several things going in my favor, I reminded myself. First, my particular therapeutic approach has always been heavily focused on using what I refer to as the *here and now*. By this I mean that the interactions the patient and I have in the moment are the essential tools of change. Whatever problematic tendencies a patient has—their insecurities, their neuroses, the things they do that get in the way of their relationships with others—these are all likely to show up in the therapy sessions, through their interactions with me. Jerry, who had to have *the best* therapist, is an excellent example. Even though he came to me for help, and thus presumably began our work with a positive opinion of me, he constantly criticized me in many ways. Time and again I brought his awareness to this tendency. At first he attributed the comments to my inadequacies, that I was overly sensitive and jealous of his financial success. But little by little Jerry began to see that he behaved this way elsewhere in his life as well, and that it impacted his relationships, and his happiness.

This here-and-now approach is largely ahistorical, meaning that it does not rely a great deal on patients' personal histories. Rather than spend substantial amounts of time digging through patients' backstories, time which I would not have in these single sessions, I focus on the present, tuning in closely to every word and gesture they offer, as well as those that they omit. I was confident this approach would allow us to get into the serious work quickly. It also had the great benefit of dovetailing nicely with the limited capacities of my faltering mind: remembering the past was increasingly challenging, and recalling copious details about each patient was beyond me. But being present *right here* and *right now*, that I could do very well.

A second thing I had going for me was that nearly all of the people who requested consultations had some knowledge of me in advance. Over six decades I have written many books, including influential textbooks for student therapists, philosophical novels, and books of stories like this one that aim to demystify the process of therapy. Through these I have had the good fortune to become a well-known figure in the field, and most of the people who had requested consultations thus far had mentioned reading at least one of my books. It was clear from most of their emails that they saw me as having some amount of wisdom and power. I took this with more than a few grains of salt, knowing that we all sometimes seek reassurance from silver-haired elders. In fact there was a small voice inside me, adolescent and rebellious, that wanted to shout out "I'm not *that* old yet!" and cancel this whole undertaking. But for the most part I was happy to play the role of guru on the mountaintop, realizing that I might be able to use the wisdom with which people imbued me and leverage that power to help them change.

Such was my state of mind as I settled into the chair in my office and opened a Zoom window to speak with Susan, a fifty-year-old schoolteacher from Oregon who was deeply depressed. We quickly greeted each other, and I explained that I would only be able to see her one time, as noted in the Facebook posting, and that I hoped to be as helpful as possible. It felt very strange saying all of this, and I think I was laying out the groundwork as much for myself as for her. She nodded, then launched into her tragic story. Two years ago, at about ten o'clock on a Thursday night, she had opened the refrigerator and noticed that the large cherry pie she'd made was nearly gone. She had planned to serve it the following evening to close friends who were coming over for dinner, but now it was reduced to a sliver of crust oozing deep red filling.

What had happened to the pie? It was no mystery: no doubt Peter, her husband, must have eaten it. It wouldn't have been the first time.

"That gluttonous slob!" she exclaimed, bursting into tears. The fate of her cherry pie was too much. The last straw. She had to be at work until 5:30 the next day, an hour before her dinner guests would arrive. She would barely have enough time to get dressed and set the table, let alone bake another pie. The disrespect!

Brimming with anger, she'd stomped upstairs and confronted her husband, who was already in bed. They argued for ten minutes. Tempers and voices rose. He told her he had always been the main support for the family (*not true!* she protested) and that he'd eat any pie he damn well pleased. She retorted that he was an obese hog who was going to gorge himself to death.

He told her to sleep on the couch and pushed her out of the bedroom, slamming and locking the door.

"Fine," she yelled. "The last thing in the world I want to do is to share the bed with a selfish glutton."

The next morning, her hard knocks on the bedroom door and loud calls to her husband were returned with silence. Finally, she and her two daughters broke into the room to find him lifeless in bed. They called emergency services, and when the medics arrived, they declared he had been dead for several hours. When police officers arrived, they sealed off the house and searched every room. Susan and her daughters were interviewed at length—clearly the police were considering the possibility of foul play, going so far as to infer that the pie might have been some sort of weapon.

"How awful," I said. "And how much have you recovered from your husband's death?"

"I'd say zero," Susan replied. "No recovery. None at all. Perhaps I'm getting worse. I miss him so much, and I am racked with guilt about what I said to him that last night. And I'm also mad at him for leaving me. I cry all the time and now *I'm* the one who can't stop eating and *I've* gained sixty pounds. I saw a psychiatrist here recently and he said that I was, in some way, identifying with my husband. What help was that? I've developed terrible skin problems and I can't stop scratching myself. I can barely sleep, and when I do, I keep dreaming of Peter. When my daughters leave for college in a month, I'll eat by myself in restaurants and people will look at me and, I'm sure, pity the dumpy fat woman eating all alone."

She caught her breath loudly, perhaps holding back tears.

"That's it, Dr. Yalom, I've unloaded on you. That's everything. I don't know what else to say."

She slumped back in her chair.

"You know, Susan, I've worked a lot with women who have lost their husbands and your account of what you're going through is not unfamiliar to me. Let me ask you something. You say your husband died over two years ago. Can you compare your condition now with a year ago? Is it different? Is it less painful?"

"No. Just the opposite. That's what torments me; I think of him more and more, and when I'm alone in the house I'm terrified of being sad and lonely forever. Damnit. It's not fair."

"Grief always lessens, but it takes time. Usually the course of grief goes through a predictable cycle. It's most keen the first year when you experience the first birthday, the first Christmas or New Year's Eve, without your spouse. But then, as time passes, the pain lessens. And later, when you go through the cycle of the special days for the second time, it becomes markedly less painful. But that isn't happening for you. Something's blocking you and I have a hunch it's related to your anger."

Susan nodded vigorously and I asked, "Can you put that nod into words?"

"I have no words for it, but I feel you're right. It's confusing. I'll be drowning in sadness and then, suddenly, all I feel is intense anger."

"Let's focus there, on your anger," I said. "Just let your mind go there and for a couple of minutes please share your thoughts with me. In other words, think out loud."

She looked puzzled and shook her head. "I don't know how to start."

"It might be easiest to start at the beginning. Think out loud about your very first encounter with anger."

"Anger . . . anger. The first time I felt anger was with my first breath—at my birth."

"Keep going, Susan."

"There was anger when I was born. My mother's anger. I remember her saying time and time again that she wanted a boy and if I had been a boy, she would have stopped there. She just wanted one child, and it wasn't me. She let me know about it over and over."

"So you spent some of your early childhood hearing about how your birth, your very existence, inconvenienced her?"

"Oh God, yes, she made me feel it all the time. Damn her for that!"

"And your father?"

"Worse. Sometimes even worse. His favorite joke, which

he never tired of telling, was that the nurse made a mistake when I was born and brought the family the afterbirth instead of the baby."

"Ouch. Oh, Susan, how dreadful to have your father joke you're not a person, that you're a placenta."

"He thought that was such a funny joke. And my mother agreed. I'll be honest with you. I know it's unnatural, but I *hated* them. Both of them. My father especially. He wouldn't pay for my college. He wanted me to work as a secretary in his store instead. So I left home early and had to work my way through school."

She paused, letting these deep emotions swirl through her. After a moment, while she was still in that open tender place, I pushed her to go deeper.

"And the anger toward your husband? Tell me about that."

"It wasn't like my anger toward my father. Certainly not at first. I met Peter after I left home, when I was in college. We were sweethearts and he was good to me. His parents were well off, and he always had money. Whenever I was strapped for cash, he'd help pay my rent or buy groceries. And I'd never had that kind of help or affection before.

"Peter's father was a politician and wanted him to follow in his footprints. Peter had the charisma—he could be incredibly charming and fun. But he was lazy, a poor student who gambled whenever he could, and eventually flunked out of school. He became a guard at a local bank, a job his father got him. He never made enough to support us or, if he did, he secretly gambled it away. Either way, he made it clear that I always had to work. I never took time off, except three-month maternity leaves when I had our daughters. I could never become my-self, never be the kind of mother I wanted to be for my girls. Instead I worked, worked hard. And you know what? Just a few days before he died, he told me he'd gotten too heavy to be a bank guard, and they'd moved him to office work, which meant a pay cut. He said it wasn't a big deal, and I got so mad at him because he didn't even care about his health. And probably I would have to find a second job to pay our bills."

"I hear lots of anger rumbling, Susan," I said. "A husband who never recognized all the work you did, who never valued *your* needs and wants. A cruel father who saw you as either a problem or a punch line. And a callous mother who never wanted you, never offered love. Now they are all gone— mother, father, husband—all gone. And a good bit of your life has gone by as well. Oh, Susan, no wonder you're angry. Who in your situation wouldn't be enraged? I know I would be."

She nodded as I spoke.

"How does it feel to hear me say that, Susan?"

"Hard. Right. But hard."

"I want to take a moment to look at all you've accomplished in spite of them: two loving children, a valuable teaching career, and so much more. You've done so well, Susan."

She swallowed, taking that in.

"I haven't really been able to talk to anyone about this," she said. "Everyone wants to remember Peter as a good person, remember us as a good couple. No one wants to talk about the darker side."

"Thank you for sharing it with me. Your anger is only human. Yet I suspect it presents a big problem. We feel we should never speak ill of the dead, that it's wrong or somehow disrespectful. Does this ring true for you?"

She nodded, tearing up.

"Well, I disagree. Anyone in your situation, with the experiences you've lived, would have the angry feelings you're experiencing. You're judging yourself far too severely."

Susan was sobbing now, and I waited for her to calm down and breathe.

"I don't know what to do, how to stop it," she said finally. "I'd like to remember so many other things about our life together. I really did love him. But now I'm just so mad."

"I suspect that as you accept your anger, accept that it is appropriate and you have good reason for it, those other memories will return. But it will take time."

"Maybe." She nodded. "I hope so."

Then, in my most solemn voice, I continued. "Susan, I've listened carefully to everything that you've told me, taken it all in and pondered it carefully. I want you to know that I pronounce you innocent. Please hear that: *I pronounce you innocent!* You deserve a good life. You've worked hard, you've been a good mother, a good wife, and you deserve some happiness now."

She smiled through her tears, and I finished the session with a keen sense of having been helpful. I gave her the name of a therapist with whom she might continue. Clearly this old man still has something to offer, I thought on reviewing our meeting!

I received a follow-up email from her a couple of weeks later which confirmed this. She thanked me for helping her, writing:

> *I won't forget the moment when you said something like "apparently your mother and your father were not good parents, but even so you've done extremely well in life . . . I admire you for that. . . ." You gave me a warm feeling of being seen and respected and supported at the same time. . . . Also your pronouncing me innocent. I will never forget that remark, and the smile on your face as you said it. I will keep the sound of your voice in my mind and my heart.*

Thinking about it later that night, I felt this was one of my best therapy hours ever. I resolved to keep offering these unusual one-hour sessions, to see whom I could help and to glean as much as I could from the process. Equally important, I would share what I learned. Earlier, speaking of my desire to help patients, I left out the other major aspect of my professional life, that of teacher. Most of my work as a writer has been in the service of teaching young therapists and others practicing, or entering, therapy. Furthermore, many of my thoughts have gone against the grain, countering major trends in the field. While psychiatry has increasingly pushed medication as the solution to mental illness, I have championed human connection; while psychotherapists have increasingly been taught approaches that aim at symptom reduction, like cognitive behavioral therapy or solution-focused therapy, I have embraced curiosity and deep personal exploration.

This dedication to sharing what I've learned has always been a powerful force driving me forward, and I began to feel that impulse again when thinking of Susan, and imagining many rich brief encounters ahead of me. I would undertake this project not only to help those who seek consultation and to remain engaged myself, but also to pass on what I learn.

CHAPTER 2

If I Could Climb Out
of That Hovel

There are some rare people, such as Susan, for whom a perfectly placed intervention or deep encounter may provide most of what they need. But I am not generally a proponent of short-term therapy, and I want to be clear that I am not in any way proposing this single-session format as a complete form of therapy. Indeed, I have long championed significantly longer-term therapy. Why? There are many reasons, most important of which is that I am most interested in helping people truly learn more about themselves, and that kind of thing takes time.

I suppose I am a therapist of big issues: searching for meaning in life, one's identity, understanding one's impulses and behavior. These goals simply can't be reached quickly in most cases. And yet the mental health fields, particularly in the United States, continue to push toward shorter and shorter duration models. This pressure does not come from a concern for better patient outcomes; rather it is driven largely by insurance companies who don't want to pay for more than eight or twelve sessions, and much prefer so-called evidence-based models such as cognitive behavioral therapy. There certainly are issues for which short-term therapies are useful, but these are often focused on very specific challenges a patient is having—trying to quit smoking, for instance, or addressing symptoms such as procrastination or avoidance. Broadly speaking, however, these short-term approaches do not do well in helping people fully understand and change the underlying causes of these symptoms. And for many people, such deeper insight and transformation are essential. My next patient was a good example. Our short time together would prove eventful, but not nearly long enough to help her address the significant challenges she faced.

Her name was Julia, and she was a young doctoral student in economics. She sauntered into my office without making eye contact and flopped down in the chair across from mine. She wore dusty blue jeans, an oversized Stanford sweatshirt, and long strikingly unkempt brown hair. It was the middle of the day, but she looked exhausted. Her eyes quickly circled the room. One wall was mostly windows, and another was taken up completely with floor-to-ceiling shelves housing the library of psychology and philosophy books I'd accrued over the previous six decades. Julia stared at the wall of books for a moment.

"You've read them all?" she asked.

"If I have, I've long forgotten most of them."

This elicited a thin smile.

"So, Julia," I continued, "from your email I know only that you're a grad student and that you've moved here recently for your studies. Tell me why you've come to see me and what I should know about you."

"To be honest, I'm not sure *why* I'm here or what I expect from you or from any therapist for that matter. I'm twenty-six and have spent well over half those years in therapy. And no one and nothing has helped."

"Yet, despite all this, here you are today requesting a consultation with me because . . . ?"

"A week ago I was at the Stanford bookstore looking at the faculty authors section. I picked up one of your books because of the catchy title, *Momma and the Meaning of Life*. I read the whole thing in one night, something I haven't done in years. I enjoyed it mostly, especially that bizarre last story, 'The Hungarian Cat Curse.'"

This might be interesting, I thought. That story is the most farfetched I'd ever written: a therapist falls in love with a woman whose family has been cursed for generations by a ferocious cat who haunts the dreams of their romantic partners. Ultimately therapist and cat engage in an exploration of philosophical ideas about existence and mortality, all over Chinese takeout. So who knew where this conversation with Julia might lead?

"What struck you about that story?"

"I don't know. But it got to me. Maybe it was the way you hung in there so persistently with an impossible patient—a surly talking cat, for God's sake. Next thing I knew it was morning, and I picked up the phone and called you."

"Something about the characters moved you?"

"I'm not sure. Well, maybe I related to that cat who had used up eight of his nine lives. I get that. Yes. I really get that cat's situation."

"You mean that you've used up most of your nine lives?"

"It sounds weird to hear you say it, but yeah, something like that. The other thing was that you seemed like a straight shooter. I've gotten so much bullshit from counselors and addiction specialists, all with their own pet strategies. I called you a week ago and, to be honest, the enthusiasm has kind of faded away now. I came close—this close"—she held up her thumb and forefinger only millimeters apart—"to canceling. I *know* there is nothing you can do for me. I am beyond repair."

Beyond repair. That was how Julia and I started.

She then launched into describing a very long line of physicians and medications and hospitalizations. Wilderness survival retreats for addicts. Meditation programs. Acupuncture and yoga. Horseback riding therapy. I'd rarely heard such an endless procession of failed procedures and failed therapists. And her manner of speaking, her defeated demeanor, and the sad indifferent way she looked at me and said "*I am beyond repair*" suggested I would soon join their ranks.

I had only one short hour to be helpful, or my name would be added to her list of failures. Worse, my failure would further confirm her sense of being irreparable, and likely make her even less hopeful for future improvement. I knew I had to act fast, but what could I do? Under other circumstances I might begin by exploring her psychiatric history further, inquiring into her childhood, and searching deeper for the root of her addictions. But I had the strong feeling this would simply waste our precious minutes together and leave Julia in that same place of despair. No, this called for something brash, something unexpected that would catch her attention.

"You know, Julia," I said, "with all you've gone through, with all the pain and suffering you've experienced, I'm shocked at how little therapy you've had. Why haven't you taken better care of yourself?"

Jerking her head up, she peered closely at me and said, "Hey, where you been? Haven't you been listening? I've just finished telling you that I've spent most of my life in therapy."

"I did hear a lot about management. About wilderness survival. About drug abstinence programs. About meditation and medication. But I did not hear one word about understanding yourself, or having compassion for yourself and what you've been through. I realize my definition of therapy may be a little unusual, but I think we can aim higher than management. I heard a lot about what you were ordered to do, but not much about what you wanted to do—what you, Julia, thought and felt and dreamed and desired. So I'll say again, and, trust me, I'm dead serious: *I am absolutely shocked by how little real therapy you've had.*"

She sat up in the chair a bit more and, as if to prove she was "beyond repair," sprung into the details of the physical and sexual abuse her older cousin and his older buddy had inflicted on her when she was a child. Then, she told me, when she was eleven, her father abandoned the family for another woman, and she never saw him again. Next it was drug use in early adolescence, trying to numb the pain. When she finally worked up the courage to tell a social worker about the sexual abuse of her childhood, both her cousin and his buddy ended up in prison, and the rest of the family stopped talking to her.

"Julia, you're telling me about major, major trauma. Hearing this, I have a powerful sense of why you've struggled so much." I paused to let that seep in, to let her know that I saw her not as a collection of labels but as a fellow human.

When she looked up, I continued. "Also, I want to note that what you have done with these crappy cards you have been dealt is extraordinary. Most people would be broken, yet you are getting a PhD at Stanford."

She nodded. "Broken, yes."

At the end of the session, she appeared disappointed when I told her again that I was retiring from practice and that she needed long-term help. I told her I truly felt she could make real progress, and I stressed to her that it was important she work with someone she could count on for the long haul, someone who could go deep with her, and not simply pre-scribe medication or some easy fix. I gave her the name of Dr. J, an excellent therapist who had been one of my very best students. I explained that she had experience with both deep existential work and more acute addiction treatment, which is a somewhat rare combination. I thought she would be a good fit for Julia, someone with whom she might make excellent progress.

Hearing this, Julia tried to appear tough, but it seemed to me her face had grown softer. As she got up from the chair, she said, "Thanks for listening so well. And thanks for trying."

Then, as she turned to leave, she said, "But, as I said before, the truth is I'm beyond repair."

I'm beyond repair. How terribly sad. I had never heard any-one say that before. I thought about this for some moments after she left, and I wished, deeply, that I could have given her more.

Soon, however, I was distracted. Shortly before our hour, I had walked out to the mailbox and received a package of paperback books, several foreign-language editions of my memoir, *Becoming Myself*. After Julia departed I picked up a beautifully printed version in a language I could not recog-nize. Something Scandinavian, I suspected: I would have to ask Marilyn when I got back up to the house. I opened the cover and began skimming through the pages, stopping to glance at some of the photos. I landed on a picture of myself as a fat-cheeked three-year-old, standing on a chair next to my mother and sister. We all seemed happy in that moment at the photographer's portrait studio.

But the truth is I had a terrible childhood. We had lived in a dangerous neighborhood in Washington, DC, above my father's liquor store where my parents worked endlessly. It was a Black neighborhood, and in those heavily segregated times I had no Black friends. If I had, my mother made it clear, they would never have been allowed into our home. And the few white people nearby? All deeply anti-Semitic, showering me with shouts of "Jew boy!" and "Christ killer!" whenever our paths crossed. I was alone almost always, left to my own devices by my parents, who spoke mostly Yiddish, while I spoke only English. I craved friendship constantly, and never received it, especially after my older sister, Jean, left home for college when I was ten. I ate my meals alone. I spent my days alone. My only refuge was the public library, my only companions its books.

Looking at that picture, I was suddenly shocked by the idea that I had managed nonetheless to live a life worthy of a memoir, one that people across the world, who spoke languages I could not recognize, let alone understand, might want to read.

I stood there for a few minutes, shaken by how unreal my own life journey suddenly seemed, when I heard a soft knock on my door. I pulled myself out of my reverie. I was not sure whom to expect, as Marilyn now rarely left the living room couch.

"Come in," I said.

It was Julia. She reentered, holding a check, and said, "Sorry. I forgot to give you this."

I thanked her and she turned to leave. But then, impulsively, I beckoned her back, saying, "I'd like to show you something." I leafed through the book I was holding and found a photo of the dilapidated building where I had lived the first fourteen years of my life. It was run-down, with peeling paint and two flimsy doors smudged with dirt and grime. One led upstairs to our apartment, the other to the liquor store. Just looking at it, eighty years later, I could remember the dank smell and the skittering sound of the cockroaches, which had terrified me every night as I slept on the living room sofa.

As she stared at the photo, I said, "That's the door to my home. That's where I came from." I intended to say more. I intended to say, "If I could climb out of that hovel, you can climb out of *your* past." Instead I was suddenly overcome with emotion. Perhaps this was because touching my own child-hood pain was simply too much just then, with Marilyn so ill and myself so diminished. Or maybe it was the dreadful trauma Julia was carrying, and the massive struggle ahead of her. What I knew for sure was that if I uttered one more word I would begin to weep aloud. And then what would we have? An old man in tears and a young woman who was beyond repair.

I think she sensed it and said nothing. She stared at the photograph for a long time, then silently mouthed, "Thank you," and left my office.

I doubted I would ever hear from Julia again yet, at the same time, I had a strong feeling that this last interchange, my showing her this picture of my dreadful beginning, might have changed her life.

The following day, she phoned and requested another session. My plan, of course, was to work with patients for only one session. But I felt I could remember Julia and the details of our session for a couple of days, and her situation seemed so dire that I agreed. Plus, to be frank, I was curious. I'd made an unconventional intervention in showing her the photo, and I wanted to see how it turned out. Yes, even at this advanced age, I am still inquisitive about my work and my patients.

What gets through to them? What helps them change? And how can I be a better therapist? Age-old questions of the field, all still fascinating to me.

When I saw her later that week, she began by asking whether I would be willing to work with her even for a short time. I repeated that I was too old, my memory too un- dependable. She turned to asking questions about what I envisioned her work with Dr. J would be like. *What would they do together?* I couldn't be sure, I said. To my mind each real encounter between therapist and patient is unique. I said I hoped they'd develop an authentic relationship that Julia would be able to learn from and grow in. I hoped it would become as safe a space as possible in which she could examine some of those dark periods without being over- whelmed by them. I hoped those terrible experiences of her youth could be transformed into parts of Julia's life, not its determining factors. I hoped that she could learn to see her strengths, see how remarkable it was that she'd thrived in many ways despite the dreadful abuse she'd suffered and the terrible shortcomings of those who should have raised and protected her. I hoped she would learn to love herself and perhaps let others give her the love she so richly deserved.

She took this in, attentive to each thought. Then she said, "I notice you haven't mentioned the drugs or the drinking."

"Obviously important. And one reason I suggest Dr. J is that she has a lot of experience with addiction *and* with exploring these deeper issues of trauma and meaning. Those issues are deeply connected, but for many reasons the approaches to treating them are often different. I believe she can help you navigate both."

My answers seemed to satisfy her and at the end of the hour Julia assured me that she would call Dr. J.

What of her feelings about my showing her the photo of my childhood home? My life-altering intervention? No mention of it. Maybe it hadn't been important to her. Or maybe she was being kind to an old man overwhelmed by emotion.

I was reminded yet again of a humbling reality. It is rarely a therapist's brilliance that makes the difference. Our clever interpretations? The bold interventions that give us bursts of adrenaline and self-satisfaction? The occasional stroke of something that feels like genius? These usually go unnoticed by patients. Instead it is almost always the qualities of the relationship, the empathy, the desire and ability to truly see the other, and the willingness to give honest feedback that one so seldom gets in regular life. These are where the treasures lie, a truth borne out in my decades of experience, as well as significant peer-reviewed research. These single hours, I noted, were likely best used to focus on the relationship.

CHAPTER 3

No Second Dates

S o much changed over the six months that followed. Marilyn had succumbed to cancer in November 2019, taking with her much of my own interest in living. Several months before she died, we had begun writing a book together, *A Matter of Death and Life,* in which we alternated authoring chapters, recording in detail our experiences and storms of emotions as her end approached. We both channeled our energy into this project, and for me the task of articulating my ideas prevented me from being overwhelmed by the sheer magnitude of my fears and sadness.

Her last days came and went, family and friends gathered for her funeral, glowing eulogies were read, and copious tears were shed. I know many close friends came to celebrate her life, but I cannot remember any of it. I fell numb, stunned into bewilderment by the loss of my love, with whom I'd been partnered, inseparable, for over seventy years. Living without her seemed inconceivable, and I often wished I could have taken her place in death. That was magical thinking, of course. But the idea of following her into the void, of ending my life—or more accurately of *having my life end* in some unspecified way—came to mind often.

How did I get through this period? I am not entirely sure. I continued to write each morning, working on the "my life after her death" portion of our book, for another four months. The writing gave me some purpose, some reason to get out of bed each morning. It also prolonged my connection with her, as her words, not yet finalized in print, seemed to keep her alive in some way. I am sure I stretched the process out, dreading what would happen when I sent off the final edits to the publisher.

Soon the COVID-19 pandemic descended as well. I began taking consultations once more, the video sessions breaking up my days. These, and regular visits from my devoted daughter, Eve, were the only things that interrupted my extreme sense of isolation. She helped me get through many of my darker days, hustling me out of bed when I claimed to be too depressed and taking me for long strolls through the neighborhood. I had lost interest in eating, so she tried to fatten me up by making sure the freezer was stocked with ice cream. And she helped navigate my continuing memory loss, keeping track of my medications and doctors' appointments, and finding movies with relatively straightforward plots and not too many characters, which we would watch together in the evenings. I got some pleasure out of that, but almost everything else had lost its shine.

Eventually it was time to send off the final draft of *A Matter of Death and Life*. The panic I had foreseen surrounding this never fully materialized, however, because my brain had already become engrossed in another project: the single-hour consultations were increasingly interesting, and helping others allowed me to focus on something other than myself. Further, every couple of weeks a session would stand out as a possible teaching story, an encounter based on which I could write a story that would reveal something unusual and useful for young therapists. Meeting with Sophia was just such an encounter.

She introduced herself over email as a single, forty-year-old trauma surgeon living in Scotland. She had emigrated from South Africa the previous year, after both her parents had died in a car accident. That was all I knew, that and the fact that I would have only one hour in which to be helpful.

We met on Zoom two weeks later, and her first comment to me was striking: "I am truly alone in the world and terrified by the thought of spending the rest of my life this way. I have no close friends in Scotland. And I am very concerned by my problems developing an ongoing relationship with a man."

"Why is that?" I asked.

"I've had a bunch of first dates, sometimes one or two a week, but I almost never have a second date. Am I hideous? Am I too stupid?"

"I don't think either of those is the problem. I've barely met you, but you are clearly intelligent, and unless you're using a very effective video filter, you appear far from hideous."

She smiled briefly.

"So let's figure it out," I continued.

"I've been in Scotland for over a year and have developed no social life at all."

"How did you come to be in Scotland?"

"The UK had a physician shortage, and I needed a change. It was too hard to be in South Africa, with all the memories of my parents."

"And your life now?"

"My professional situation is good. I enjoy my hours seeing patients, being hands-on effective in crisis circumstances. On weekends and nights I do research, which is satisfying. But my social life? Zero."

I pointed out that she had recently moved to a new country, and right before a global pandemic began, which was a significant and unusual barrier to developing personal connections.

"Not a huge difference for me. The hospitals are still open, so I'm with people all day at work. Plus we'd all be in surgical masks, anyway, COVID or no COVID."

"And the move doesn't feel significant?"

"I didn't have many friends in South Africa either."

I made a mental note that her challenge went beyond romantic relationships, which might be significant. Then I went on to explore her life in the same manner that I had successfully used with countless patients—although sped up a bit given the circumstances. But somehow each attempt I made to draw her out resulted in a deft deflection. She responded amicably to each question but only with simple, surface-level responses. She didn't seem to want to explore any of the avenues I proposed and withheld any deep personal information.

After fifteen minutes of this, I began to feel quite distant from her, which is often my cue to move into the here and now. The first step was to shift our focus from her difficulties relating to others in her life to exploring what was transpiring between us in our conversation.

"Sophia," I said, "let me ask you a question. How are you and I doing today in our session?"

"I've not spoken to a psychiatrist before. This is my first time."

"Can you say more? Tell me, what is it like for you to speak with me?"

"As I said, I've had no experience with therapists. You're the very first. But I'd say we're proceeding properly."

Faced with another conversation-terminating response, I told Sophia I was experiencing real difficulty connecting with her. I wanted to know what was going on inside her but felt uneasy. She appeared interested in my comments in the abstract, but when it was time for her to respond she continued to be stingy, offering as few words and as little disclosure as possible.

I tried to focus on her emotions, thinking she might need more direct prompting. "How do you *feel* about the questions I'm asking, Sophia? What emotions are coming up for you?"

"I'm not clear why you keep asking questions about how you and I are doing. It seems entirely irrelevant to my reason for contacting you," Sophia said.

"Not at all," I said. "Let me explain what I think is happening. First, please try to think of our meeting today as a social microcosm of what goes on with you in the real world."

"Social microcosm?"

"I mean that, to a great extent, the way you interact with others is being replicated right now in your interaction with me. As I understand it you're an intelligent and attractive woman who meets many men for first dates, but for some reason they never contact you again. That's the mystery I am trying to help you solve. I believe that by examining our relationship—that is, what you and I are experiencing right now—we can find the answer."

She seemed to ponder my words carefully, then nodded again but did not respond.

I leaned in a little closer to the screen. "Let me share my honest personal reaction to you in our session so far."

Her eyes opened wide in an apprehensive look of surprise

that nearly always follows when I make this offer. I believe this is because most of us never get truly honest feedback from others. Instead people's responses are invariably colored by the type of relationship they have with us, such as high emotional stakes with lovers, or status with colleagues. But offering such honesty is one of a therapist's most powerful tools.

"From the very onset," I told her, "I've been trying hard to get to know you, to get closer to you. We only have a little time, so I'm eager to do this as quickly as possible. That's why my questions are quite intimate. But I am making very little progress. You appear distant and ill at ease and, whatever I ask, you give me little of your personal feelings. I feel in a bind. I want to help you open up, but I also feel awkward pressuring you so much. Am I being clear?"

"So, you're saying that this very meeting with you right now is a social microcosm?"

"Exactly."

"Hmm, that's an interesting way to put it," Sophia said. "Okay. Let me try to be more open. My answer to your question is that I feel a bit flustered and a bit annoyed with you."

"Great! And I suspect that what happens here in *our* discussion is very similar to what happens with you and others. Are you with me?"

"That I get annoyed with others?"

"Perhaps when they try to get too close."

She nodded, more engaged, and I continued. "Now, Sophia, can you take a risk and tell me more of your feelings about our meeting so far? Try not to hold back. Don't worry about offending me."

"Well, you say 'don't hold back,' so I won't. Here is *my* honest response. There's a piece of me that is frustrated at how incessantly you're pushing me to open up."

"Can you keep going?" I said in a calm, inviting tone.

"Sure. This is getting irritating. You are getting irritating! No, let me rephrase it: I am irritated and, if this were a normal conversation, I would have walked away quite some time ago."

I nodded, indicating she'd hit on something important.

"But I haven't walked away because . . . maybe I'm beginning to grasp what you're saying. The truth is I don't open up. I'm not used to it. And I'm not comfortable doing it. Why should I?"

"Now we're getting somewhere," I said. "I think this sheds light on your critical question: *why no second dates?* Imagine the person you are out on a date with, okay? They spend the evening trying to learn about you, trying to see if you are someone they want to open their hearts to. But every time they try to get closer, you deflect their questions. After a couple of hours and maybe a drink or two, they come away feeling pretty shut down, convinced that you aren't very interested in them. Maybe they don't merit your attention."

She nodded slowly, taking this in. I could sense she was wrestling with the implications.

"I understand opening up is uncomfortable," I offered. "But you may need to stretch out of your comfort zone if you want someone else to get close to you."

"Okay. That won't be easy for me, but I'll have to try . . ." Her voice trailed off. Clearly something else was troubling her. After a minute she continued, "So it's my fault . . . all these people, all these missed opportunities?"

"You've played a part," I said, "but only a part."

I let that sit between us for a few moments. Then I shifted gears, knowing that too much self-blame wouldn't be helpful. A sense of responsibility can be very helpful in inspiring change, but self-flagellation rarely is.

"What do you know about the origins of your discomfort?" I asked. "Where did it come from?"

"I imagine it goes back a long way. My parents were missionaries and were quite closed off, and I was brought up that way."

"How so?"

"Their work was important. And it was important to them that I checked all the boxes—did well in my studies, behaved well, and represented their position in the church and the community."

"Sounds restrictive."

"Very."

"And emotionally? For instance, if you were upset about something?"

"There was not much space for my problems."

We had run over the hour, but it was time very well spent. Sophia appeared to have grasped the concept that both her outside behavior and inner feelings had been replicated in our interaction, which allowed her to see what she was bringing, and not bringing, to these many first dates. This was one of the numerous hours when I felt sad that I had come to the end of my tenure as a therapist seeing patients over the long term. Sophia was primed for change, which is always an exciting moment. I would have loved to work with her. But, alas, like Sophia, I am having only first "dates" now, these single sessions with patients. For her, that is a problem I think she is now on a path to altering. For me, I suppose, these first dates are a temporary solution to the intractable, inevitable problem of my aging and memory failure. How would my "date" respond, showing up for a second encounter only to learn that I have little memory of the first? They would likely feel rejected, as if they or their problems were so insignificant that they didn't merit my attention, even when they were paying a significant fee for it. This would certainly not be conducive to building the warm, close relationship successful therapy requires.

But I think I have been helpful to Sophia, which isn't half bad for a first date.

Two months after our session, I sent her this story and requested permission to publish it, as I did with all the patients in this book. I received this response:

Hello Dr. Yalom,

It was so nice to hear from you. Truthfully, my experience during our session was as uncomfortable as yours, especially for the first half-hour, but then it improved, and ended with some relief. You pushed me considerably, which I am not used to, and that made me very anxious. At points I was annoyed and even angry. However, our meeting served me well, and I have continued to think about my contribution to my relationships, or lack thereof.

We talked about my parents as a source of my challenges opening up. Since then I've realized there is another thing that holds me back. You may remember that I am a trauma surgeon, so I often see death, and people facing loss. For instance, a few weeks ago a bearded man in his fifties was wheeled in on a gurney after a horrific motorcycle crash. The worst are always motorcycles. I did my best to patch him up but he was in bad shape with lacerations, broken bones, hemorrhaging. It could have gone either way for a while. When I checked in post-op he was still out cold. A woman, his wife, sat holding his hand. She'd been crying, and I could feel her anguish as soon as I came into the room. I think caring that much about someone terrifies me.

Someone who could be gone in an instant. How could I bear the pain? And yet I hear a voice inside (yours?) telling me that to truly live I must be willing to risk loss.

I rely a lot on my dreams, especially the feeling I have upon waking, for answers regarding my life. After our session I was prepared for an unsettling night. On the contrary, I woke from a dream with a very warm, sweet and calming feeling. I took that as a good sign, and I had the strength to tell a man I am interested in that I wanted to see him again. He admitted to being surprised, but pleasantly so, he assured me. We are having dinner this weekend.

Thank you,

Sophia

One reflection about this encounter, which is critical to therapy in general, and here-and-now work in particular: several times during the session Sophia noted how uncomfortable it was for her to talk about what was happening in the space between us. This was no surprise. In our regular lives we rarely talk in this way. Most of our conversations are filled with what therapists call *content*: this is what happened, how we responded, what happened next, etc. But with Sophia I was insisting we talk about *process*, that is, the dynamic between us, the patterns of communication, and the emotions that arose and were expressed or avoided. In normal life such direct process talk often feels uncomfortable, even disrespectful, perhaps because we are having our subtle behaviors examined in minute detail, and being held accountable. But here, in therapy, this type of close examination is extraordinarily useful.

In Sophia's case the *content* she presented—her lack of friends both in Scotland and previously in South Africa, her parade of unsuccessful dates, her loneliness—all related to interpersonal distance. Investigating our *process*—the way she deflected all my attempts to learn about her and engage her on a personal level—revealed a dynamic through which she unintentionally contributed to the negative outcomes she described. This clearly suggested that to address the problem she would need to put down her defenses, to open up more if she wanted people to get closer to her.

CHAPTER 4

Colonization, or Showing Off

In the weeks that followed I thought often about Marilyn's death, and my own. I had dreaded her passing immensely, with an aching apprehension that had made any pleasure nearly impossible for months. But now I was surprised to realize that anxiety about my own death, a palpable angst that had plagued me throughout my life, was barely present. It was odd, almost disorienting, to feel largely free of this familiar fear. I suppose this shift was due to losing her, and to my ever advancing age. By the time I was eighty-eight, nearly all my closest friends were dead. I felt like the last wrinkled leaf clinging to a branch in autumn. Without Marilyn, there were no emotional bonds that strongly tethered me to the living. My children were dear to me, of course, but they were all deeply engaged in their own lives. It brought me joy to see them, but I had also begun to feel like a burden at times. They would miss me, as would a handful of friends and students. But given my age, the sadness that would come with my passing was close on the horizon.

There was another, less gloomy element that freed me of much death anxiety: I have been fortunate to live a rich, full life. I didn't feel I had a lot of unfinished business. The end was in view, but much less frightening than I'd expected, or that I feared it would be for many, many years. It wasn't until I was directly confronted with it that I felt at ease with dying.

In 1980 I wrote a book called *Existential Psychotherapy*, bringing together many thoughts about death and mortality, the ways this aspect of the human condition impacts us all, and how to use an existential lens to work with therapy patients. Put very briefly, we all live in a uncertain world and are confronted by a number of inescapable givens of living, which I categorize as: *Death* (we can only live fully while aware that we will inevitably die), *Freedom* (we have enormous freedoms and are ultimately responsible for our own life choices), *Isolation* (we are born alone and will die alone, and yet desire intimacy and merging), and *Meaninglessness* (we exist in a confusing world where no absolute set of values exists, and yet we crave meaningful lives).

While many of the clinical approaches to working with these concerns came out of my own observations, the book is rooted in the work of great philosophers, authors, sages, and others who have long pondered death and how the specter of dying changes our living. Twenty-five years later I revisited these themes in *Staring at the Sun*, looking at how to overcome the terror of death, and again drawing on the wisdom of great thinkers from the classical Greeks to contemporary philosophers. Clearly these concerns have been central in my own thinking, and my work on them has been influential for many therapists with similar leanings.

My next consultation was with Christine, a young therapist who was drawn to the existential approach. I had received the following email from her:

Greetings Dr. Yalom,
I'm a psychiatrist who has just finished residency and am now
starting private practice in Oregon. I'm a devout follower of
yours, particularly your existential work. I saw your Facebook
post a few weeks ago in which you stated that you are now
offering a supervisory session via Zoom. I would very much
like to schedule an appointment with you.

Christine L.

Obviously Christine had misread my Facebook posting in which I had used the term *consultation*, not *supervision*. *Supervision* has a specific meaning in the field and entails taking a mentorship role, reviewing the therapist's cases, and having some ongoing responsibility for the therapist, and potentially their patients. Given her existential focus, her interest in my supervision would make sense, but it was a much different proposition than I'd offered, and certainly more than I could provide.

I replied that I'd be pleased to see her for an hour's *consultation* and offered some possible dates. She emailed me immediately, stating that she'd be delighted to have some *supervision* from me and we settled on a date and time. I noted, but did not comment on, her persistent use of *supervision*.

In longer-term therapy, gathering a patient's initial information when we are together in our first therapy session can be an opportunity to glean insight. What aspects of their life, for instance, does the patient deem most important? What things might they gloss over but subtly hint they hope I'll pick up on? What areas do they seem to avoid? But at this point, eight months into my single-session experiment, I had learned subtle exploration was inefficient in such a limited time span. Getting as much information as possible beforehand became very useful, so a week before my appointment with Christine I wrote back, asking what particular issues she would like to address in our hour consultation. She responded that she had just completed her training and could benefit from my supervision as she entered into private practice. Yet again I noted her continued use of that specific, professionally laden word. I did not know where this might lead, but I suspected that she might have trouble relating on a personal, rather than professional, level.

We began our Zoom session and my first impression was that she was both highly intelligent and very eager to speak, as if she'd been holding back a great deal, waiting for this meeting.

"Thanks for seeing me, Dr. Yalom," she began.

"Call me Irv, please," I said, seeking to quickly close the distance between myself and my patient.

"Okay. I have to tell you that this is not a great time for me."

"What's happening in your life now?"

"Well, as I mentioned in my email, I've recently finished my psychiatric residency, and I'm having a rocky start to my practice."

"Rocky how? Tell me about that."

"I've got my office. I've hung up my sign. Furniture, plants, website? Check, check, check. But I don't have patients other than the few I took with me from my residency. They won't keep the lights on, that's for sure. I have yet to get a referral from any members of the faculty. Not a single one!"

"I'm sorry to hear that. That's got to be unsettling. Any ideas why?"

"Oddly enough, *you* are part of the reason."

"Me! How so?"

"I've been a Yalom follower for some time. I've read all your books, many of them more than once, and I consider myself a disciple. I'm particularly drawn to your thinking on existential problems, how death anxiety impacts us, how we all must grapple with the shadow of death and meaninglessness in our lives. Well, the faculty members in my psychiatry department often presented their long-term patients to the students, so I've heard dozens upon dozens of treatment plans. But none of them ever mentioned that idea of death anxiety. Not once. They're ignoring the very core of therapy!"

She paused, clearly expecting me to join in her irritation.

"Existential work often makes people uncomfortable," I offered. "Therapists included."

"Well I kept quoting you, and that just annoyed them, and made things worse."

I was flabbergasted. This was a first for me. In all my years seeing patients, I had never been the cause of their problems— not before I'd met them at least! It is not unusual for patients to be upset with their therapists, usually because they attribute thoughts or attitudes to us, as if we think poorly of them or don't care about them. I have certainly had patients upset with me for all sorts of reasons. But I've never had a patient begin our time together this way. There was a part of me that wanted to dig further, to learn more of her thoughts about my work, perhaps how I was viewed by her faculty and how I had impacted her. But this was my own ego speaking, as it often does, and the therapy was about her. I turned instead to focus on her experience of this seeming rejection by her professors.

"Christine, I get the idea that you must have felt very isolated and perhaps uncared for in your training."

"True. Very true," she said.

"Tell me, what kind of work did you do on this in your personal therapy?"

"Wow. That was quick. You've hit on a hot point. I've never had any ongoing therapy."

"Really? I've written a good bit about how important it is for every therapist in training to get their own therapy. Tell me, why haven't you?"

"I know, I know. And I did try. I started twice and quit twice. The two shrinks I saw were both hopelessly rigid. The first one was unbelievably pompous. His walls were covered ceiling to floor with books, all with overly complex, polysyllabic titles. In one session I pretended to be interested in one of the books and asked him about it. He wouldn't answer. Or couldn't. Just covered up. I suspect he had never opened the thing. The other therapist I tried was obviously intent on colonization and I terminated after only a couple of sessions."

"Colonization? Curious word. What do you mean?"

"Oh, Dr. Yalom, you know. It's your word: you used it often in *Existential Psychotherapy*, which is sort of my Bible!"

This stumped me for a moment. I had no recollection— zilch—of using this word. And yet it seemed so obvious to her, a phrase I'd used *often*, one that had clear meaning and importance. How strange, to have this young woman tell me about my own idea, and not be able to recognize it. I felt un-moored for a moment, exposed and vertiginous. I consciously chose not to follow that train of thought, not to give in to that feeling and use our time to relieve myself of my own discom-fort. I anchored my attention back to her.

"This is a little embarrassing, Christine, but I can't re-call using it. My memory is spotty these days, and no doubt you're right. I'll have to look it up. But let me make sure we're on the same page. Do you mean the therapist will somehow invade your psyche and take possession of you?"

"Precisely. Couldn't be better put."

"So, let me be sure I fully understand. The first therapist

was fraudulent and the second was invasive. Tell me about other therapy you explored."

"That's it. Never was willing to take the risk. I'm proud of who I am and I don't want to be tampered with."

Tampered with. Interesting word choice. I made note of it, then moved forward.

"I imagine that did not fly well in your residency. Personal therapy is a requirement in all psychiatric training programs I know of. I wonder if you tend to avoid examining problematic areas."

She shook her head in consternation. "Now you're losing me entirely, Dr. Yalom. How could you possibly assume that from the few minutes' discussion we've had so far?"

"It's evident in the emails you sent me. Do you still have them on your computer?"

"I'm sure I do."

"Check them out when you have a chance. In your first note you remarked that you read my Facebook post announcing that I was offering *supervision* sessions to therapists. But, in fact, my Facebook post said I was offering *consultation* sessions. We had two more email exchanges and each time this exact pattern was repeated. I used the word *consultation* whereas you insisted on the word *supervision*. Since I made that post on Facebook, I've received several hundred requests for sessions. Yours was the only one that changed the word *consultation* to *supervision*."

"I'm sorry but I'm still lost."

"Sorry to be so indirect. The point I'm trying to make is that there may be a lot of meaning in your preference for *supervision* rather than *consultation*. To my mind consultation implies a need for help, which would require telling me about your own serious concerns. Supervision, on the other hand, implies professional oversight, that is, looking at how you deal with other people's concerns. I'm guessing that your reluctance to use the word *consultation* is because you feel uncomfortable opening yourself up, looking at your own issues."

"Yes, now I'm following you. And you're right, that is on target. I just had no idea it was so obvious."

"Well, I've been doing this for a while. My sensor for these things is pretty strong—even as my eyes and hearing are fading."

She was clearly engaged, right there with me.

"I wonder, too, if that is the reason that the faculty isn't sending you patients?"

"Because?"

"Maybe they can sense that you need to do more work on yourself, work that will make you more welcoming to potential patients."

"What do you mean?"

"Well, I think one's comfort with oneself, and honest knowledge about one's biases, is critical to therapy—and readily apparent to patients."

"Apparent to patients how?"

"Whatever their specific problem, patients are struggling. They are seeking someone whom they feel can help guide them, someone mature, whose presence is calming. If they sense that you are unsettled, that may leave them ill at ease."

She pondered this idea for a few moments, then nodded. I hoped she was weighing the idea of getting into personal therapy and deciding in favor.

Watching her, I suddenly had the strong impression of her need to prove herself, and to resist authority, almost like a teenager rebuffing her parents. I began to ask about this, even as some part of me knew I shouldn't.

"One more guess," I added. "I'm sensing a problematic relationship with some older person. Your father? What was that
like?"

Christine seemed startled and hesitated before responding.
"Whoa. I was with you until you asked about my father. That's
spooky. I didn't tell you anything about my parents. Uh . . . I
don't know what to say."

I took in her shock and realized I had gone past what was
most helpful for her. I read people pretty well, but this must
have felt like divination, given that neither her father nor any
other relationships had come up in our conversation. I could
imagine her feeling like she'd come for therapy consultation
and gotten a psychic reading instead.

"I'm sorry, Christine. That was a misjudgment on my part. I
knew I was going too far, but I couldn't stop myself. I just felt
strongly that you hadn't had a good relationship with your father and that your experience with him was an important factor
in your deep caution when you interact with your teachers and
therapists."

We sat in silence for a few moments. Eventually I said,
"Christine. Let me ask you a question I often ask of my patients.
How are you and I doing in this session?"

"Hmm. I'm having such a swarm of uncomfortable feelings,
I'm not sure I can dig into this. I feel kind of frozen."

"I think I've overloaded you. Tell you what, Christine, let's
try something different. Okay?"

She looked at me puzzled. I had pushed a bit too far and
made her feel uneasy and less likely to engage in our process
together in a trusting, open way. I switched gears here to bring
her back by being as transparent as possible about my own
thinking and my own mistakes.

"My question to you was: *How are we doing in this session?*

I'll pretend you asked me that question and I'll try to answer, okay? I think we were making good progress in our meeting, getting to know each other a bit, and identifying that you struggle with opening up for fear of others taking over, colonizing you in some way. I pushed further, with the observations about *supervision* instead of *consultation*. This shook you a bit, but in a useful way, I think. So far so good. But then I screwed things up with my guess about your father, which really wasn't necessary. You were already getting the point—about how your avoidance impacts your work as a therapist—but I just couldn't resist showing off how clever I was, and now I feel a bit embarrassed. Showing off is an old problem of mine. I've worked on it for many years, but it still keeps popping up. Please forgive me."

"Are you being serious?"

"Indeed I am. That is truly what's going through my mind. Christine, can you try to respond?"

"I'm a bit stunned by what you just said. You want honesty, so here goes. I don't think I have ever had a conversation like this. Talking so . . . really saying what I think without worrying so much that the other person will be offended."

"And yet we're both alive and kicking. We're surviving. We're closer and more honest with each other. This is what I want for you. It's essential to experience such deep and honest work, first as a patient and then as a therapist."

"Right, my getting personal therapy. Honestly I think I'm just fine as I am. And I really don't want anyone tampering in my head."

"Do you feel like I'm doing that with you now, tampering?"

"Well, no. You have surprised me, kind of like you've gotten inside my kitchen and tinkered around. But not in an invasive way."

"And?"

"It feels like we are connecting, like I can be open with you. Particularly since you admitted to showing off."

It's funny how often my missteps provide excellent openings. Once again I was reminded that being present, sharing myself as a full and flawed human, always seems the most helpful position—much more so than being an unreachable expert.

"I think this open communication is the way therapy should be," I said. "Not tampering. Think about it from the perspective of your patients: you are asking them to open up, to explore their emotions and their most challenging dark corners. It is essential that you know, through your own experience, what you are asking of them, and what you are offering—which is ideally this very transparent, honest engagement. Therapy, good therapy, is not about invading the other but helping them discover themselves.

"Alas, the clock is telling us it's time for us to wind up. I'm sorry we have to stop, but I want to encourage you to do this work for yourself. As soon as we end our session today I'll email some names of colleagues who would work well with you— none, I think, who are colonizers. How does that feel to you?"

"Mixed. So many feelings. Scary. But I trust you. I'll try to do it."

"I'm sorry I can't instantly populate your practice," I said. "But this is much more important work. You will discover many things about yourself and, I'm certain, become a better therapist as a result."

I have written at great length about the importance of therapists getting personal therapy elsewhere. If Christine is indeed a "Yalom disciple," then no doubt she has encountered these thoughts. But knowing that something is helpful and actually doing it are quite different, as anyone who has tried to break a long-ingrained habit can attest. Especially if one has a trepidation of the change, such as fearing a therapist will somehow take over one's inner workings, as Christine clearly felt. I hoped she would take my exhortations to heart.

To be an effective therapist you must both understand the experience of therapy from the patient's perspective and get to know yourself extremely well. This last piece is critical to working in the here and now, because you need great awareness of your own perceptions and biases. During the session, a good therapist is reading the interaction and making careful notes of the emotional responses they are having to the patient. If, for instance, I find myself getting frustrated at a patient's evasiveness, as I had with Sophia of the first dates, I need to recognize that I'm having this frustration immediately, rather than sinking into the emotion without awareness, as one usually does. My frustration indicates something critical about the interaction we're having, in this case that Sophia's refusal to open up was off-putting to me and, by extension, likely to others she encountered. If the therapist has blind spots about themselves, then those emotional responses will not be reliable indicators of how others would generally respond, and the idea of therapy as social microcosm falls apart.

Imagine, for example, if in the midst of a session a patient is complaining at length about his wife, and the therapist notices herself getting bored. This is important information that may indicate the next direction for fruitful digging. The therapist must trust her own perceptions and suspect that others will be similarly bored by the way the patient perseverates and casts blame elsewhere. She may do well, then, to suggest the two of them look at what has happened in the space between them, leading to discovery about how, for instance, the patient uses a complaining attitude to cast himself as the victim in his relationships, pushing away those in his life who might listen.

This is the here-and-now dynamic when it functions properly. But it only works if the therapist is aware of his or her own blind spots. Imagine if the therapist above had been in a marriage that ended poorly, and in which she felt unfairly blamed. If she were scarred or resentful from this experience, and had not done the work to identify her own bias, her ability to use herself as a delicate emotional detector in therapy would be skewed. Imagine also that the patient mentioned above actually had very good reasons for complaining about his wife—perhaps she belittled him constantly, often wishing out loud that she had married her now successful high school boyfriend. The therapist might, once again, be put off by how the patient seems always to complain about his wife, and suggest that this is the patient's key problem. But now the therapist might be wrong. Her negative response might be a result of her frustrations about her own divorce, which she has never worked through.

We all have unconscious biases and neuroses that might make our perceptions less reliable, and more fraught with potential countertransference. Knowing oneself as deeply as possible is essential, and exploring one's faults, strengths, and dark corners as a therapy patient is the best way I know of honing one's perceptions in service of providing one's patients the most effective therapy.

Some hours after our session ended, a thought I had avoided dwelling upon seeped back into my mind. *Colonization.* The word echoed in my mind. *Colonization.* I had no recollection of using this word. It seemed almost foreign, unrecognizable.

And yet Christine had been sure it was an essential concept of mine, a word I used *often*. How strange, to think someone else might know my work better than I do. And yet this is an irrefutable aspect of my aging. My daughter often knows better than I if I've taken my medications on a given morning. And friends have reminded me of trips they claimed we took together years ago, but which I cannot recall. Perhaps, I thought, it should not surprise me that this would be true of my writing as well.

This thought provided a brief wry smile, but no comfort. I reached for a well-worn copy of *Existential Psychotherapy* on my shelf, the one I had used when lecturing on countless occasions, thinking to search for this word. I opened the cover and was greeted by notes scribbled in the margins with several different colored pens. I noted page corners folded over, flipped through and found marked passages, and more and more notes. I shut the book in a bit of a panic. This task suddenly struck me as ridiculous. I was in no condition to reread my major works. I'd get lost in no time, my mind buffeted in one direction and then another. Occasionally I have picked up one of my books, most recently the comedic novel *Lying on the Couch*. I'll read a couple of chapters and have only the vaguest memory of the characters and plotline. It is confusing! Plus I often come away with the bittersweet thought: *That guy I used to be, he is a really good writer! I wish I could write like that now.*

I put the textbook back on the shelf. And yet *colonization* stuck with me, and with it an uneasiness that my own life, being reflected back at me, was unrecognizable. I went to my computer and did a search through my files—that much I could manage. Next I sifted through a file cabinet of very old notes. I even called one of my colleagues and asked if they remembered my use of this idea. Ultimately I found one brief mention of *colonization*, not in *Existential Psychotherapy* but in another book of mine, *The Gift of Therapy*. There I used it as one of several reasons people might avoid intimacy in their lives, which I followed directly with the suggestion of caring therapy *as a corrective emotional experience*, in other words as an anecdote for this block to closeness. I felt a wave of relief. I had not "often" used this word. It was not a core concept of mine that I had since forgotten, as Christine's assertion had implied. I was not yet so unrecognizable to myself.

Then another thought crystallized: each reader is going to bring their own issues to whatever they read. In Christine's case, this was the fear of somehow being invaded and taken over by a therapist, and perhaps by other close relationships. Regardless of whether this notion of colonization had ever been a major idea for me, it was certainly one that resonated loudly for her, and was thus transformed from a relatively minor idea (to me) into one of great import (for her), which she *knew* I had used often. The point here is not how often I actually used it (and in fact I could be wrong; perhaps were I able to reread *Existential Psychotherapy* I would encounter multiple instances), but that each person has strongly subjective experiences of life, and therefore of reading. These experiences color our vision, causing us to focus on certain things rather than others, and to respond emotionally to different things in distinct ways. This is true of all the patients one might see, and it is true of therapists as well. Coming full circle, this subjective focus is precisely why therapists need to be as aware as possible of our own responses and biases, and why we *must* undergo significant personal therapy. Whether or not I recognized *colonization* as a core idea of mine, the response I gave Christine came from a deep-seated theoretical stance, one that had not yet succumbed to my memory loss. I was still me, still working in a way that was true to my beliefs about psychotherapy. And while some of these one-hour sessions have shaken me a bit, ultimately my approach has held up again and again, providing a familiar comfort within the work and reaffirming the power of connection between therapist and patient.

CHAPTER 5

Like a Comet Completing
Its Orbit

An email arrived from Paul, a young gay man in Arkansas. He was desperately unhappy, he explained, for reasons that piled one upon another, reenforcing his sense of hopelessness: a terrible rupture with his parents, the bitter end of a romantic relationship, his sense of deep isolation and shame. For the past several months he had been seeing an elderly therapist who had been helpful but who was now retiring. Ironically that therapist had referred Paul to me, as if I were a younger and more vital alternative.

Paul's lengthy email struck me with its string of extraordinarily complex yet graceful sentences. It began:

I am a 22-year-old government employee living in Arkansas, not the most propitious of beginnings. Needless to say, it is a long way, both geographically and, I suspect, culturally, from my town to yours, and during ordinary times this chasm would have prevented me from sending this missive. However, with the plague postponing all face-to-face contact indefinitely, from these Southern backwaters to the haloed intellectual halls of Stanford University, I hold out precious hope that written correspondence might enjoy a brief renaissance.

In reading your work, I often find myself moved not only by the dedication and sensitivity with which you approach each of your patients but by the universality of your insights. More than once, I've read past what I take to be a "bespoke" revelation, derived from a singular encounter with a particular patient, only to experience it returning to me in some seemingly distant aspect of my life several days later, like a comet completing its orbit.

What an image! And I'll admit the lofty praise made me feel good. A few lines later Paul wrote:

Dr. Yalom, it occurred to me that, with civilization as we know it on hiatus, you may now be conducting consultations over the phone or video. If so, then the distance between us will have more or less collapsed and, barring the probable existence of a full schedule on your part and what I can only imagine is a waiting list longer than the Bayeux Tapestry, it mightn't be so foolhardy of me to hope that I might arrange a private appointment with you.

Indeed, it was not foolhardy, I thought with some delight. I did have a waiting list but only of several weeks. I was booking just one consultation each day, which took all the stamina and focus that I could muster. This single-session adventure had opened many new opportunities. It gave me windows into many different lives, amplifying what has always been a pleasurable aspect of my work. I very much looked forward to a quick "visit" to Arkansas, and to an hour spent with Paul of the long, eloquent sentences.

On the morning of our session, I finished a cup of coffee and slowly walked to my office. It was July 2020, four months into the COVID lockdown, eight months after Marilyn's death. The last vestiges of spring were still holding on, and delicate blossoms from the few gnarled apricot trees remaining of the orchard that had once covered our yard dotted the gravel path. Inside I turned up the thermostat and sat at my desk. As always, there were several books piled beside the monitor. Post-it notes were stuck around the desk as well, jotted reminders of this idea and that, which had proliferated as my memory had become less reliable. I shuffled several books and notes off to the side, clearing the space so I could more easily focus on the screen. I glanced again at Paul's email to refresh my memory.

Moments later his face appeared, and my first impression was of a delicate, shy young man who seemed almost apologetic for disturbing me. Seeing me, a gentle smile flickered across his face. His voice had a slight lilt to it, and his speech was confident, just as poised and arresting as his written prose. That was on the surface. The *content* of the session, however, turned out to be shocking and sad.

When Paul was eighteen, he told me, his parents, with whom he had had a close, loving relationship, learned he was gay. They cut him off immediately and had neither spoken to him nor supported him financially, or in any other way, during the four years since. At an extended family gathering the previous year, in fact, his father had avoided his gaze, pretending not to see him. This brutal rupture had shaken his world completely. Their cruelty and neglect was so extreme that I was surprised he had done as well as he had, finishing college and finding work to support himself.

As I listened to him recount the extent of his isolation, his feelings of hopelessness, and his deep sense of not deserving anything from life, I felt uncertain about what I could offer him in this one hour against this enormous litany of struggles. Over a longer course of therapy we could have built a powerful alliance, learned where these self-defeating thoughts had come from, assessed them in light of our present relationship, and together worked on connection, and on his self-image. It seemed likely that many of these negative feelings arose from guilt or shame around his sexuality, a clash of values inflicted upon him by his parents and the conservative religious culture in which he grew up. Examining both the devastating rift and the restrictive assumptions of Southern manhood would feature prominently. But there was no time for such work. With only one hour to battle against deeply engrained beliefs I listened differently, seeking a more radical approach, something that might jar him and loosen the grip of these pernicious dogmas.

Time and again he repeated, in one way then another, that he did not warrant better than his sorry lot: that he was an abomination for loving men, or that he was pitiful for not boldly defending his love for men, that he had squandered the intelligence and privilege he'd been born with, that he was simply worthless. I pondered how best to respond when, suddenly and without my cooperation, I heard myself asking an unexpected question: "Tell me, Paul, what are you writing now?"

Paul froze, his face entirely puzzled but suddenly alive. He opened his mouth, but no words came. He shook his head.

I persisted. "Let me ask again: *What are you writing now, Paul?*"

"You got me," he said. "What do you mean? I'm baffled."

"The email you sent was extraordinary. It left me astonished. Over the years I've received countless messages from readers and potential patients, but rarely have I gotten a letter written in such superb prose. You're obviously very gifted. Hence, my question, what are you writing now?"

He was alert, more present and engaged than before. What he said next sounded like an apology.

"I do set pen to paper at work I guess. Office communications for the Department of Agriculture. Exceedingly boring. There's no creativity involved there."

"And how long have you had this job?"

"Three years. It pays the rent. I guess I think it's all I deserve—and all I can do."

"And when you're not working?"

"I'm fully occupied with two projects: feeling sorry for myself and cursing the meaninglessness of existence."

The meaninglessness of existence tugged at me, as well as the idea that a dead-end job was all he could do. I noted both, perhaps to return to later in the session, but persevered on the point of his writing.

"Listen to this," I said, and read from his message. "You, Paul, don't simply remember insights. Instead you experience them returning to you *'several days later, like a comet completing its orbit.'* Magnificent! So help me understand this conundrum: you have been given this rare and glorious talent that sits unused. *Why aren't you writing?*"

Paul didn't know. The vigor that appeared when I mentioned his writing was there, but so was a weary sadness.

"I guess I don't take myself seriously. At times, wonderful sentences make brief appearances in my daydreams. And often I imagine the first lines of stories and novels. But they never linger, nor proliferate."

He tried to go further but could not, and sat silent for some time. He shifted to speaking of the many things that he had worked on with his therapist: his two-year relationship that had just ended, the loneliness that lay ahead, and his deep shame about his effeminacy, which was compounded by living in Arkansas, a state not known for its progressive views.

I responded to each of these concerns as best I could, but none of these elicited the spark of vitality that had come over Paul when I mentioned his writing. Near the hour's end, I returned to that more fertile area with an unusual suggestion.

"It's very rare for me to recommend a TV series to a patient," I said, "but I urge you to watch *Anne with an E*, based on the novel *Anne of Green Gables*."

"That's your prescription, Doctor?" Paul asked with surprise.

"Bear with me. I'm in the midst of it right now and I'm entranced by the extraordinary young teenage star who is similar to you in that she, too, speaks in delightful, elaborate sentences—"

I noticed my hand reaching for something on my desk. What? A Post-it note upon which some words of dialogue were scrawled.

"Here, I jotted these lines of hers down several days ago," I continued, surprised that my hand had found exactly what my mind was racing for. I read, "*People laugh at me because I use big words, but they are exciting and descriptive words, like* enraptured *and* glorious. *If you have big ideas, you have to use big words to express them, haven't you?*'

"As I watch the remaining episodes, I'll continue to think of you and your graceful phrases and sentences, Paul. I also urge you to continue therapy. Immediately after we end our session today I'm going to email you some good referrals, excellent therapists who work on Zoom. I'm particularly thinking of one

LGBTQ+ affirming colleague who I think will provide some insight and inspiration for a struggling young gay man."

That shy smile I'd seen at the session's outset flickered across Paul's face.

"And I want to say once more, it is time to take yourself seriously and to start writing. Trust me, I've spent most of my life writing and reading. I recognize talent when I see it. I hope you'll take my observations to heart. My goal right now is to help you avoid the deep regret that you will experience if you reach the end of your life without attempting to become what you might have been."

"Message received," Paul said. "Loud and clear."

"And one last request, Paul, a favor really. Please send me a finished piece, one that pleases you very much."

"I give you my word, Dr. Yalom. I shall do that."

As I think about what transpired in my session with Paul these many months later, I can only point to what must be some sort of intuition that prompted me to ask what he was writing. It's not that Paul had in any way stated explicitly his desire to write. But his depressed affect seemed so distant from his passionate language, and it was clear that he felt trapped in what he saw as a hopelessly mundane government job, his spirit wasting away at a young age. It has been my experience that when people resist an important life force, it often leads to intense feelings of hopelessness. When there is something you know, deep inside, that you must be doing in the world, and yet you are prevented from doing—by fear, shame, parental approbation, financial need—it can take a heavy psychological toll.

During our short session these thoughts did not come to

me consciously. Rather I acted on unexpected impulse to ask about his writing. Perhaps the impulse surfaced because I've been at this so long, and perhaps I chose to follow it because the urgency of these one-hour consultations has led me to be bolder in my choices than I might be otherwise. Whatever the case, when I asked about his writing he instantly became more alert, more engaged. Some passion and desire had been touched, which helped shake loose the frustrated and helpless feelings. For him, as with many others, some validating feedback about one's excellent traits goes a long way. I left this encounter very eager to hear from him, and to see what progress he'd make. I very much hoped that my explicit support of his writing would nudge him out of the dark rut he found himself in and help him pursue his literary impulses. Most important, I hoped he would follow up with the therapist referral I'd sent.

A few weeks later I sent Paul a draft of this story and requested his permission for publication. His response:

I must say how touched I am that you've adapted our encounter into a story. I am delighted to offer you my permission to publish it. After all, it's been a lifelong dream of mine to be seen by the world as an effeminate 22-year-old homosexual from Arkansas!

I promised to send you a completed story, and I sorely wish that I could attach one. However, I do have two pieces of good news. First, I've found Dr. G, whom you suggested, to be an excellent therapist and, indeed, an excellent human being. I'm extremely grateful to you for connecting us. You were quite right in your intuition: it has been helpful to have a gay therapist, and one whose obvious joie de vivre is a constant advertisement for how happily a gay man might embrace his authentic self. I also credit him with reminding me of how fine a hobby it is to play piano. I can't say I'm a very proficient instrumentalist, but no matter—whenever I sit at a keyboard, I'm emboldened by a line from The Importance of Being Earnest: *"I don't play accurately—anyone can play accurately—but I play with wonderful expression."*

Second, I have been writing much more than I usually do, which means that, unless I lapse into an unprecedented stretch of laziness, I should be able to send you something before too long. I find that writing in the way that draws on my innate voice is an activity I can only seem to manage when I've achieved a certain state of equilibrium. What I suppose I mean is that, if I ever teeter toward depression, as I'm afraid tends to happen with alarming regularity, the first warning sign is almost always the near-complete evaporation of my ability to write coherent sentences. It's as if all my words are restless citizens, and I the maligned king they desperately hope to overthrow. Heavy lies the head that wears a crown, Dr. Yalom. Until then, I hope that you remain in high spirits and robust health.

In gratitude,

Paul

CHAPTER 6

Memory, Ah Memory

I thought a great deal about my session with Paul in the weeks that followed. I was delighted by our connection over writing, for him because another fine writer might now have inspiration to get words on the page, and for me perhaps because I no longer have Marilyn with whom to discuss literature, and conversing with Paul filled that need for a day. Yet there was a moment in our session that left me bewildered, not as a therapist but as a human being struggling with aging. When I mentioned the delights of *Anne with an E*, my hand sought out the Post-it note upon which I'd written some lines of dialogue from that show. It was truly acting without my conscious instruction, or even knowledge. In fact, I'm certain that at that moment I was unaware of having written that note, let alone that it was nearby and might be beneficial to share with Paul.

Of late, I have been watching my mind carefully, aware that my brain is changing and my memory deteriorating. I grow more alarmed and ashamed as reminders of my forgetfulness appear every day. Where is my cell phone? Did I lock the doors? Oops, I left the oven on overnight. Have I already seen this film or read this book? The characters seem vaguely familiar. And did I remember to ask Eve to bring coffee beans when she next comes to visit? I could call her, but chances are good she'll say, "Dad, you just asked me to do that a couple of hours ago." It is relentlessly distressing, leaving me feeling both infantile in my capacities and reliance on others, and alarmed by my decline. Nonetheless, I've made a habit of staring directly at this deterioration. I've spent many decades working with my patients' mental and emotional struggles, and the brain and mind fascinate me. Now I have the chance to observe its aging process from the inside, and I find myself intrigued in spite of the pain and embarrassment.

So just what was going on with this hand and this piece of paper? Slowly, old memories of my medical neuropsychiatric training drifted back to my mind. I began to recall, faintly, the difference between explicit and implicit memory. *Explicit memory* is at play when we occupy ourselves with such things as studying for an exam and retaining facts and faces. It is clearer and more intentional. *Implicit memory*, on the other hand, is not conscious. It relates to feelings, muscle memory, and familiar patterns like navigating your way around the neighborhood you've lived in for years. Learning music theory, for instance, relies on explicit memory, while strumming chords on the guitar you have played for decades engages implicit memory. Neurologists have done copious research on these two forms of memory, and there is considerable hard evidence that they are formed through different pathways and reside in two very different sections of the brain. From the outside perspective, how curious, how exciting. From the inside . . . how strange. I unconsciously remembered having stuck that Post-it note to the side of my desk and found my hand reaching for it: *implicit memory* on full display. As my explicit memory continued to flake away, it was good to know this wasn't the whole story.

It was an August morning, a few weeks after my eighty-ninth birthday, and I was employing a tried-and-true way of jolting my explicit memory: I was rereading the email I'd received from Elsa, with whom I was going to meet in thirty minutes. Clearly, I had not read her message carefully enough the first time, for I was surprised to discover that she had seen me for several sessions of therapy ten years previously. Yikes! I had no recall of her whatsoever, so I scrambled to find my old session notes. If things had gone according to plan when I had seen her back then, a clear protocol would have been followed, and there should be a neatly labeled folder in the file cabinet beside my bookshelf, filled with clearly typed notes. For many decades after seeing patients, I would walk around the yard outside, dictating session notes into a small microcassette recorder, which was the height of technology at the time. I would hand these cassettes off to Bea, my wonderful longtime secretary upon whom I was completely reliant, and she would deftly transcribe them so I had organized records of my many patients.

Unfortunately what I found that day was quite different. Elsa's folder was there all right, but inside was a cluster of lined yellow notepad paper, covered with dark scrawls parading as handwriting. Uh-oh. Bea had died ten years earlier, and for several months after her death, I had handwritten my notes until I began using a computer dictation program. It must have been during those few months that I had met with Elsa. I have had terrible handwriting since I was a child, and becoming a doctor had been license to keep it that way. My notes were disgracefully illegible. All I learned from looking them over was that Elsa and I had met for a half dozen sessions, and that she was having such major marital difficulties that she had been on the brink of divorce. At least so I thought: I could make out the words *divorce* and *affair* and *children*. Somewhat clearer was a sentence stating that she had cherished my support and had asked for a hug at the end of our last session. And then, lo and behold, there was a printed email she'd sent following that session, in which she noted that the hug had been important to her and had served as an antidote to her father's and her husband's coldness and cruelty. There was something to work with, at least.

While I was anxiously deciphering all of this, the time of our meeting had arrived. In fact, I was already five minutes late and received a message from Elsa telling me she was waiting. I held my breath, sent a Zoom invitation, and a few seconds later was staring at the face of a woman in her forties with high cheekbones, striking green eyes, and chestnut-brown hair falling well past her shoulders and out of the video frame. In the past, if I saw the face of one of my former colleagues or patients, a torrent of memories would pour into my mind. No longer. I did not recognize her face in the slightest, nor could I recall a single moment of our therapy together: no hug, no cruel husband, nothing.

As a therapist, I'm committed to being honest about the feelings I experience in the here and now, and have exhorted countless students to do the same. That honest willingness to offer how you truly experience the patient, and using that information as a powerful ingredient of change that you and the patient can examine together, is critical to successful therapy in the here and now. Suddenly I was facing an enormous challenge to this core value: How could I possibly tell Elsa that I recalled almost nothing about our previous sessions? She had expressed such gratitude, such strong and positive feelings about our connection, that I feared she would be deeply hurt to know how little of her I retained in my memory. I wanted to avoid inflicting such pain. My mind raced for alternatives. I could lie, assure her I had a clear recollection of her, and attempt to bluff my way through. Such a dishonest encounter seemed equally unacceptable.

Which path to take? I mulled over my guiding principle: What would be in her best interest? It wasn't clear. Flustered, I settled for a rather muddled approach, attempting to avoid all mention of not remembering her. I justified this decision to myself by arguing that I could still offer her something of value. I would focus on her current situation and, as best I could, sidestep any mention of our earlier meetings so as not to detract from the real opportunity for positive work together now.

Then a very odd thing happened. As I continued looking at Elsa's face, I experienced a strong rush of warmth toward her. I did not recognize her, nor did I feel a flood of memories return from our session. But I felt intense positive emotion, a keen desire to be helpful, and a powerful sense of protectiveness. Though I could recall almost no *explicit details* of my previous meetings with Elsa, the *implicit warm feelings* that I had toward her were obviously very much alive and well preserved somewhere in my mind.

Of course I often have positive feelings toward my patients, and meeting with them generally brings me pleasure. But this potent wave of emotion was quite different, almost as if my emotional system were compensating for my lack of conscious awareness. It was surprising, and briefly disorienting in a pleasant way. How odd, to feel so strongly toward someone with no recollection as to why!

Elsa seemed pleased to see me and launched into telling me that things weren't going well, and she was worried that her children were struggling. Cautious, I asked some gentle questions, hoping her responses would trigger my memory. Unfortunately my brain remained obstinate, and I remembered nothing. For a moment I felt anxiety mounting. Soon, however, I became aware that every remark I made seemed to soothe her. It was clear that she was benefiting from our conversation, even if I were not as specific or insightful as I would ordinarily have been. Somehow just encountering me had allowed her to release some tension. And seeing this positive effect allowed me to do the same with my fears of not being helpful. For whatever reason—presumably a positive role I'd played at an earlier stage of her life—being with me was something of a salve for her. Overall this was not the ideal beginning for a therapy session, but it was a place to start.

She began to fill me in on the years that had passed. When we'd seen each other last, she and husband, Ted, had been fighting constantly. She was frightened and confused—this hadn't seemed like the man she'd fallen in love with and married.

"There was an affair?" I offered, remembering the scrawled notes I'd written.

She looked away, and I wished I hadn't said that. What if I

were wrong? Things had been going well between us. Had I just messed it all up? Would she see through me, suddenly realize I had no idea who she was?

"I thought so at the time," she said, turning back to me with a sad smile. "To be honest I still don't know. He just changed so much that seemed likely. Maybe."

Okay, I thought. I'd gotten away with that one. No more overly ambitious guesses to show I remembered her. I would just stay present and engage fully in what was happening.

"Do you have any other ideas about what changed?"

"I think it was the kids, mostly. By the time Charlie, our third, was born, it was as if Ted resented me. He took every opportunity to make nasty little comments here and there. I did think there must have been someone else—we certainly weren't having sex at that point. Then a great job opportunity opened up for him in Boston, and I thought moving away might break whatever was going on."

"And?"

"There was a brief period when things changed. He even . . . this is a bit hard to say . . . he was—"

"Take your time, Elsa," I said, again having the impulse to soothe her.

"He began to be interested in sex again. It even felt exciting, to be intimate like that. But whatever that shift in him had been, it was still there. What seemed like intimacy wasn't. Sex got aggressive. Not really violent, but he wasn't sharing it with me. He was angry and taking it out on me. And I let him."

"I'm so sorry, Elsa."

"I haven't really told anyone this."

"How does it feel?"

"Embarrassing. But safe to tell you."

"It's okay," I reassured her. And again, something relaxed in her expression.

"It's a relief to say that out loud," she said, wiping away tears.

"How are things now?"

"I finally had enough and divorced him."

"Good for you, taking care of yourself."

"I'm married again, to Lawrence. He's lovely, and we're lovely together. But the kids are still caught between me and Ted. That's why I contacted you. It's a mess, and I think they really need some therapy. I didn't know where else to turn."

The kids' situation that she described was indeed a mess. They split their time between the parents, but it was a minefield. Ted had weaponized the divorce, and missed no opportunity to blame Elsa for a thousand perceived transgressions, even as he and his new wife negotiated having newborn twins. Co-parenting was fraught and draining, and Elsa tried not to engage in the emotional warfare, focusing on being present and available for her children rather than triggered by Ted's slights. But the kids were stuck in the middle, and she could see how confused and unsettled they were. I suggested two Boston-area child therapists for her children, confident that any well-trained therapist would insist on seeking changes to the malignant relationship between the two family systems.

"Thank you, Irv. It's so good to be with you again," Elsa said as we signed off.

I was much relieved at the end of the session, as my fears about repercussions from not remembering our earlier encounters proved unfounded. But this felt a bit like luck rather than an affirmation that it is not important for therapists to remember their patients' stories! If Elsa had been someone else with different needs or expectations, being with me in my current state might have been highly upsetting rather than soothing.

I am reminded of the important fact that therapists have many patients, while patients have only one therapist. This is an inherent inequality, which can sometimes be used to the benefit of the therapy—that is we *want* to be important in the patient's mind, so that our words and the experiences we share in therapy can have a powerful transformative impact. On the other hand, imagine the potential damage for someone who, placing great importance on the approval of their therapist, finds themselves completely forgotten.

In the future, I thought, I would prepare a little more carefully, making sure to note any previous connection I'd had with patients. If I did not remember someone, I would try to suck up my pride and let them know up front, trusting that being honest and attentively helping them with any resulting disappointment would be better than pretending I remembered things I did not. It seemed that this would be a better outcome than having a patient terribly upset, hurt that I did not remember them, and either being furious with me (manageable) or assuming it was somehow their fault that they were so unmemorable (potentially damaging).

Fortunately for both of us, neither of these happened in that session with Elsa. Rather, our clearly positive feelings toward each other had carried the day. To appease my curiosity about the end of stories, I urged Elsa to email me a couple of months after our session, to let me know how things with the children were progressing. Her response to her aging therapist was lovely:

Dear Irv,

I misunderstood your request for an email, thinking that you wanted to schedule another session to discuss the last one. I am chuckling at myself: obviously my misinterpretation has everything to do with how hard it is to say goodbye to you. In our session I told you I had contacted you out of concern for my children. That's not the whole truth—I suspect I also used that excuse to reconnect, not only for them, but for me as well.

I want you to be able to retire, and I appreciate that age and memory make practicing psychotherapy difficult. You should know that I feel so happy I got to see you again for our virtual session, and that I feel really good about the entire experience, including this email.

Months later I overcame my embarrassment about my memory loss and sent Elsa this story of our meeting, requesting her permission to publish it. She immediately responded:

Hi, Irv,

This description of our session is accurate and clear. I am honored for you to include it. About your memory. Yes, I was aware that you didn't recall all the details of things I spoke of. Yet this never bothered me. Not once. I always felt cared about, and your forgetting small things had little impact. This is curious to me, and I have examined myself to see if I am feeling hurt but hiding it. I have not discovered any discomfort! When I think about my early relationship with my impossible dad who scrutinized and remembered everything, it makes sense that your memory gaps coupled with your insight and care don't cause hurt.

Ultimately things worked out beautifully for Elsa, and for myself. Her deep thoughtfulness and generosity toward me were certainly part of that, and gratifying personally. Perhaps best, this encounter has given me a new insight about aging. If it was the great warmth and sense of protectiveness that I unexpectedly felt toward Elsa that set the stage for healing, can I perhaps credit my implicit memory for this success? On the one hand, some manifestations of implicit memory are unsettling—my hand reaching for the Post-it note unbidden— because they seem so out of my control. On the other hand, these experiences, and a good deal of research, indicate that implicit memory is far less susceptible to the ravages of aging, and even dementia, than explicit memory. It is common to forget faces, names, words, but still feel deep connection to people, know the words to a familiar song, or how to ride a bicycle. As my explicit memory loss continues apace, perhaps I might learn to rely on my implicit memory a bit more, view it not with suspicion but relief, and trust it when it surfaces, as it did with Elsa.

CHAPTER 7

Sparring with Serenity

Maya's face startled me. She was disarmingly beautiful, with dark reddish hair and green-gold eyes. Her smile was radiant, with a glow that seemed to reach out across the decades, bringing me back to my own youth for a moment. Ah, to have the feeling of immortality once again! She exuded a peaceful serenity from my computer screen, and I found myself somewhat off-balance, which was surprising. I am rarely so thrown by appearances and noted my response, wondering if her beauty startled others as well, and perhaps altered how they responded to her. I have worked with multiple patients for whom a beautiful face proved to be both a blessing and a curse, eliciting unwanted attention or special treatment, adulation from some and resentment from others. Both extremes skew normal interactions, and I suspected this would be relevant to our session.

I was still formulating a first question when she launched right into her reasons for contacting me. Obviously, I was not the first therapist she had seen.

"I'm twenty-eight. I've been with Charlie since I was twenty-one, and I expect to marry him. But he is getting fed up with my preoccupation with Gilbert."

"Who is Gilbert?" I inquired. "And how long has he been in your life?"

"About three months."

"And he is?"

"I got him soon after he was born."

Curious! Was her evasion intentional?

Maya seemed delighted, and watched my confusion for a moment with an almost playful expression.

"Gilbert is my dog," she finally explained. "He is the light of my life. And that's my problem right there." Maya sat back in her chair. She appeared relaxed, with no trace of concern. Perfectly at ease.

"Fill me in. What's the problem?"

"It's obsessional thinking. And sometimes behavior. It's been my issue as long as I can remember. For years I obsessed about food, couldn't stop thinking about it. So I measured every gram of carbohydrates, every gram of fat that passed through my lips. I weighed myself constantly. That's pretty much all I remember from college, really. No great books. No wacky antics with friends. Just *How much did I eat?* and *Am I still beautiful?*"

"And what about now?"

"Now my obsessional thoughts are different—although that took a lot of work and a number of therapists, and a few not entirely inaccurate diagnoses of OCD and eating disorders. But now I obsess about Gilbert. Here." She showed me a picture on her phone of her holding a small gray-and-white dog wearing a blue collar. "He's just so cute! I can't get him out of my mind. I worry about him all the time. *Is he eating enough?*

Is he lonely all day when I'm gone? I go to class, and all I think about is poor lonely Gilbert. I know he needs to have another dog for company."

"And Charlie's attitude toward your dog?"

"I'd have to say, 'Not good. Not good at all.' Charlie works hard and has very long hours—he does commercial real estate. When he comes home, he's beat. I *know* he needs downtime, I *know* he needs my attention. But I absolutely *can't not talk* about Gilbert. I just can't. *Is Gilbert happy? What do you think, Charlie? He doesn't look happy. He's alone too much, by himself for hours at a time. He needs a friend. Shouldn't we get another dog to keep him company?* I know I should be thinking about my classes and about Charlie and about our future but, instead, it's always Gilbert. It's just so hard to think of anything else."

Her words were telling me that she was concerned, that she could not escape invasive thoughts, that there was danger there. It made sense. But her demeanor was serene, a simple beatific smile playing across her face. The dissonance was striking, and I felt sure it would prove important in the hour to come.

"My mind just goes on and on. Poor lonely puppy waiting for me," she continued. "*Of course* he needs company. Every living creature needs company. And Gilbert is just so small and new to the world. And so loving, and every day he must think I've abandoned him."

I had asked her about Charlie, and she had deftly steered the conversation right back to Gilbert, our conversation bearing out the pattern of her obsessive thoughts.

"And Charlie?" I redirected.

"Most of the time when Charlie gets home, I can't wait until he takes his coat off before I start talking about Gilbert. About how lonely he must be, and—"

"Maya, let me interrupt you. Let's really focus on Charlie for a moment. How does he respond to all of these Gilbert thoughts?"

"Charlie is a kind, sweet man. He listens, and he truly cares for me. He doesn't say it, but I believe he's running out of patience. I know I talk too much about Gilbert and about my fantasy."

"Your fantasy?"

Now her face truly lit up, glowing with youth and joy. "My fantasy, my dream for the long term, is to move to this gorgeous forest area, just a couple of hours away from here."

"Tell me more," I said. "What do you imagine your life will be like there?"

"Well, I'll have nine or ten dogs. Gilbert would love it! He'll be jumping up and down with happiness and it will all be perfect."

"Perfect?"

"I mean I know we'll live happily ever after. Me and Gilbert and all the other dogs!"

I took this in for a moment. Her youthful smile suddenly seemed more naive, less glorious. Something seemed off. I grew up in the inner city and have never felt entirely comfortable out in the wilderness. Perhaps the strong negative response I was feeling was this bias? I examined my own thinking for a moment. Certainly one could live a wonderful life out in the countryside, even if it didn't appeal to me. That wasn't it. It was the "happily ever after" that struck me as so strangely detached. My mind went to how she'd teased me at the beginning of our session, letting me imagine Gilbert was another man rather than a dog. Perhaps this was more of that playfulness? Maybe she was just joking.

"It will be beautiful," she continued earnestly. "Tall trees, dappled shade, puppies leaping and scampering about. So happy."

She appeared to be entirely serious. I started to feel concerned.

"And Charlie?" I asked. "Does he share this fantasy? How would he find work in real estate in the middle of the wilderness?"

"Reality, reality, I know! But Charlie can come with me. It's not so far away, just a couple of hours."

"So four or five hours of commuting daily?"

"Or he could spend part of the year here, working, and spend the rest of the year with me."

That serene smile never wavered. If Charlie was already struggling with her obsession with Gilbert, it was clear there was no real place for him in this new vision. How could she not see that?

"And do you think Charlie will be happy with this arrangement?"

"He loves me. And he'll see how happy I am, how happy Gilbert is."

"And that will be enough for him? Enough companionship, driving hours to see you every once in a while? You did say that you love him and plan to marry him?"

"Oh yes. I know it will work out."

The more I pushed, the more committed to her vision she became. She believed her words. And she appeared truly excited about this fairy-tale future. Perhaps it was my lack of imagination, but I simply couldn't see how this could work without her relationship imploding, and who knows what else in her life falling by the wayside.

I pressed harder. "Maya, could you describe the typical day you imagine out in the woods?"

"I'll be happy with the dogs all day. I love training dogs. We'll take long walks, run around in the woods. Gilbert will be delirious. Sheer heaven."

"What will you do for work?"

"Train more dogs! And maybe some remote web design. Easy-peasy."

"And your evenings? Every evening alone, at least when Charlie's not there?"

"Well, that would be a bit of a problem. I'd probably use a lot of alcohol. When I'm alone I do tend to drink." She paused for a moment, with an almost pensive look on her face. For a moment I thought she would suddenly see the dissonance between the happily-ever-after fantasy and the real-life demands of her relationship, of her drinking, of having a satisfying life beyond the dogs.

Instead she turned back to me with a glowing grin.

I looked carefully at her face and again saw no worries, no concerns—only that unwavering smile. I felt as if we were living in two different realities, seeing the same set of circumstances in completely different ways. The scenario she described spelled probable disaster to me and perfect delight to her. Many of us seek out serenity, a calm disposition, and contentment in our lives. But I've learned that, paradoxically, too much serenity on the surface often indicates a denial of deeper problems. It can be a potent avoidance strategy. I wondered how far down Maya's self-deception went. At some deep level I felt she *must* be aware of the looming danger.

"Okay," I said, thinking I would play out a thought experiment with her, so she might see the probable results of her fantasy. "Let's look at this together. Let's imagine this all goes the way you've described it. Every day, Charlie needs to commute many hours to work so that you can live in the forest with your dogs? Does that sound right?"

"I'm sure it will all work out."

"You really don't see a problem?"

She shook her head and continued smiling that glassy grin.

What planet was she from? I thought. How should I proceed? I noticed that I was unusually hesitant to confront her and trouble her supremely calm demeanor. This suggested to me that others who knew her, her friends and loved ones, might also find it hard to be honest with her about her relationship. Apparently no one had done so yet, and I realized it was now my unpleasant responsibility.

"I want you to hear something," I said. I pulled up the original email she had sent me and read aloud:

> *I constantly seek reassurance that I am beautiful and young as though it gives me some sort of immortality or importance. . . . I worry sometimes that I'll look back on my whole life wondering why and how I let myself waste it. This is why I'd love to work with you, Dr. Yalom—I believe you can help me find a way to not let my obsessions consume my future.*

"I'm struck by your words in this email, Maya. You're making some important observations and I take your thoughts very seriously."

She nodded and continued smiling.

"I want you to pay careful attention to what I'm about to say. I think you are in great danger at this moment. You've been with Charlie for many years now. You say you love him and that you expect to spend your life with him. But from where I am sitting, that seems extremely unlikely unless something radical changes. You tell me that each night when Charlie comes home, exhausted from work, the only thing you can talk about is Gilbert—how lonely Gilbert must be, what Gilbert needs, how guilty you feel about not doing enough for Gilbert. I'm going to be very direct with you. This relationship is not going to last. The idea of living in the forest with ten dogs and Charlie is, I suspect part of you realizes, deeply improbable. You tell me that Charlie cannot work in the wilderness and that he is not interested in dogs. Forcing him to commute four or five hours sends the clear message that you value him less than you value your pet. I can't see anyone remaining in that relationship, and I doubt Charlie, however much he may love you, is the exception. So where would that leave you? Alone in the wilderness with ten dogs and a bottle every night. Is that truly the life you want for yourself?"

Maya's smile finally faded.

I waited a few moments. She did not respond. "Here," I continued, "let me read these lines again":

I worry sometimes that I'll look back on my whole life wondering why and how I let myself waste it. This is why I'd love to work with you. . . . I believe you can help me find a way to not let my obsessions consume my future.

We sat silently together for several moments and then Maya, her face solemn now, spoke. "I'm a bit stunned by what you've just said to me, Dr. Yalom. Thank you. I've been waiting for those words. I needed to hear them. I consider your comments to be tough love."

"Yes, I think that is right," I said. "Think of it as a wake-up call."

"What do I do?"

"You'll have to find your way through the emotions and give your real priorities precedence over the obsessional thoughts."

"How?"

"It will take more than one hour, but fortunately this is something a good therapist should be able to help you through. I'll do some investigating and send you contact information for a couple of excellent psychologists in your area."

I ended the session with mixed feelings. *I'm rarely so confrontational*, I thought. *Had I been too harsh? Was she ready to hear this?* One thing I was learning is that the effort to be truly helpful in these single-hour sessions often involved enormous time pressure, pressure that necessitated I make choices I would not otherwise, choices that don't follow the same logic as my accustomed therapy. In Maya's case, I resorted to a very direct confrontation, whereas generally it is far more effective to lead patients toward making these discoveries for themselves. As therapists we lay out possibilities and ask thought-provoking questions that often cause patients to consider how they are living, whether their actions align with their values, and whether their beliefs are serving them well, understanding all along that deep change has to come from within.

There is a difficult irony here because patients usually come to therapy in significant distress. What they want in that state, by and large, is a solution to the suffering they are experiencing, whether the problem appears to be external or internal. And this solution, they often imagine, is advice about what to do. But again, real change needs to come from the patient reconsidering their own tendencies and making a shift rather than being told what to do in a given situation. Almost always there is a lot less utility in my telling someone what to do rather than helping them overcome whatever internal obstacles they have so they can reach their own conclusions that better align with their deeper values.

But I was learning that there was little time for this in-depth process in most single sessions, particularly with someone as committed to her delusions as Maya was. In retrospect, I had attempted to let her see for herself how incongruous her fantasy life was with having a happy relationship with Charlie. I assumed the dissonance would shake her from her serenity, but it hadn't happened. Instead she'd responded, "I'm sure it will all work out!" So I'd given her a more direct shock by reading her own words to her and expressing my strong feeling that Charlie would not remain with her, a second-class citizen to her dogs. My uncharacteristically blunt words shook away her placid smile. Hopefully it would inspire her to get further sustained help. A follow-up email from Maya bore this out:

Dr. Yalom,
Please know that I did not feel unsettled at all by your words. On the contrary, I did not want our session to end. I don't have many people in my life who are truly honest with me. It felt liberating to hear you say out loud what I've feared but what no one will say.

You instilled a sense of urgency: I need to figure out how to be in my relationship sooner rather than later. I trust your expertise enough to know that if you fear for my future, then I should too.

A few weeks later I mailed her this story and requested her permission to publish it. She responded:

Reading this, I felt jolted again by the realization that I have been jeopardizing my relationship with Charlie. I even told him what you had said, and he did not deny the severity of the situation.

I laughed out loud at your wondering what planet I am from. I can't usually see how absurd my thinking is, but this made it clear. With the help of the therapist you suggested, I have decided to re-home Gilbert. I am devastated and I cry many times each day. Now I obsess over what it means that I can love a being so much and give him up. Still, I am thankful that our session enabled me to distance myself from my short-term fixation on Gilbert and focus on the importance of my long-term relationship with Charlie.

Part of me wants to scream that you've sucked the joy out of life. Why shouldn't I have a fairy tale? A happily-ever-after, with puppies frolicking as the birds chirp in the meadow? But you're entirely right about Charlie, and prob-ably many other close relationships. I love the idea of the puppies being so happy, but I do not want to live life alone, with wine as my primary non-canine companion. Still, on my sad days I shall think of you as "fun's executioner."

With gratitude,

Maya

CHAPTER 8

Invasione and Aggressione

I am a sociologist from Italy working to complete my dissertation while, in my spare time, trying to better my understanding of societal and global conflicts between/ within generations. I would very much love to discuss with you:

- *the departing of veteran generations*
- *views on the generation at hand*
- *the possible lack of psychotherapy and psychoanalysis in the future*

All of the above is a part of fulfilling my dream of reaching the analysts and authors who have inspired me the most in my life and career and, in time, attempting to illuminate the above-mentioned to the public.

Alberto sent me this email several days before our session, after I had asked him to let me know what, specifically, he wanted help with. I read it once. Then I read it again. There was something interesting here, but it was baffling. I found myself curious but also confused as to what he wanted. After a couple of more times reading it through, I decided the lack of clarity was probably an issue of his writing in English, rather than his native Italian. I was confident we'd be able to work it out when we met.

Alberto's intense bespectacled face soon popped onto my screen, and he began speaking immediately.

"Dr. Yalom, it is my profound pleasure to make the acquaintance of such an influential and august thinker and human."

"Thank you, Alberto."

He spoke English with a slight accent, which I found charming. I commented on this, and he informed me that he had a gift for languages and spoke five quite fluently.

"It was my good fortune to study my field in New York City, where I received a master's degree before returning to my native land in pursuit of greater specialization and socio-political knowledge."

He continued, making some observations about his program in New York, I think. But something was off. I was having difficulty hearing Alberto. I turned my computer's speaker up, but the problem persisted. I felt I was missing things he said, and I asked him to repeat himself several times. Perhaps I would have done better with my hearing aids in place, but I felt reluctant to ask for time out to locate and insert them. *How foolish*, I thought. *Here I am at eighty-nine years old, speaking to someone I will never encounter again, and I am too vain to ask for a time-out to put in my hearing aids! Would I never grow up?* I saw the humor in this but was too flustered in the moment to enjoy it.

Reason won out. I asked him to pause for a moment, and I quickly put in my hearing aids. His voice was now loud enough, but I still could not hear him distinctly; I asked whether his audio was working correctly. He nodded and pointed to the headphones he was wearing. I wondered if I should start using headphones and, for a moment, I thought of inquiring about the brand he was wearing but dismissed it. He had not come to me to give product recommendations after all but to get help with something serious in his life. I turned my attention to his narrative.

"Tell me, Alberto, how can I help?"

Rather than bringing up the grand questions he'd posed in his email, Alberto began speaking about problems with his girlfriend, Emma.

"We have shared a home for the past year, bolstering one another in this time of pandemic and intertwining our personal journeys appreciably. Yet I am uneasy, she is uneasy. Our continued future together is perhaps described best as murky."

"Murky how?" I inquired, trying to parse his rather formal way of speaking. "Say more."

"Also I am struggling to relate to my mother these days. Perhaps it would be helpful for your comprehension and assessment of my circumstance to know that I lived with her for several years after my father, may he rest in peace, passed away."

This session was not going well. I simply couldn't understand much of what he was saying. And I didn't know why! I heard his words and sentences but somehow not what he was trying to say with these words and sentences. Ten minutes passed, and I was right on the verge of ending the session. I thought of what I might say. *I'm terribly sorry, but the audio is so blurred that I'm missing too much of what you're saying. I think we should cancel our session.* Something like that. And, of course, I'd offer to return his fee.

But I didn't say this. For one, he'd want to reschedule, and then where would I be? But more importantly, I knew Alberto had been waiting to speak with me for many weeks. He clearly had many things he wanted to say. He was an intelligent man and was making a great effort to communicate. I gritted my teeth and listened harder.

I began to realize that I could hear every single one of his words. It was not that the audio was malfunctioning, but something else entirely was going on. I simply could not follow his thinking. What did his outpourings of words actually mean? They seemed so jumbled.

While trying to listen, I was also scanning distant memories of my training. The phrase "word salad" came to me. Curious. It was followed by the distinct face of an unshaven man seated in a plastic chair. Who was he? After a moment it came to me—this was a highly troubled man who had been part of an inpatient group I'd led many years ago. Why were these two thoughts colliding in my mind? Then it clicked. *Word salad* is a term for the rambling, incoherent speech symptomatic of certain types of schizophrenia. Perhaps Alberto was schizophrenic? But no, I have worked with many schizophrenics before, and his affect was completely different. And his language seemed much closer to making sense.

Suddenly a truly frightening thought gripped me. Perhaps it was not his capacity for speech that was limited but my capacity for comprehension. My own thoughts were clear, but I could not understand what my interlocutor was saying. There is a word salad phenomenon on the receiver's end as well, called Wernicke's aphasia, which can be caused by stroke and makes it hard to recognize meaning. Had I suffered a stroke? Was this to be my here and now? At eighty-nine years old, trapped in my own brain, hearing others' speech as a jumble of only partially comprehensible sentences? I felt a powerful anxiety grip me.

"What do you think, Dr. Yalom?"

Alberto's voice brought me back. I took a deep breath, tamped down my panic, and focused again on the screen. *Help the patient*, I told myself. *Help the patient.*

"Alberto, can you tell me more about the important relationships in your life?"

"Emma and I have been together for two years. Ours is the most significant bond I've ever experienced."

"Do you have difficulty conversing with her?" I asked.

"Major difficulties," he responded. "She often, very often, says, 'I simply cannot have a clear rational conversation with you.'"

Ah. Perhaps the communication problem was not all inside my head. What a relief! I felt tension flowing out of me, and breathing came more easily.

I inquired about his other intimate relationships. He mentioned a childhood friend who now lived in another country and with whom he was no longer in touch. He tried to explain the reasons for their estrangement, but I couldn't parse them. All of this was so strange that I began to wonder if, rather than schizophrenic, he were perhaps autistic. But no, he obviously wanted to connect, with me and with Emma, and he had no trouble following any of the social cues in our conversation.

The situation was ripe for here-and-now intervention in many ways: there was clearly something about the way he related that was preventing me from connecting with him, and it appeared to do the same with others. But I hesitated, because there was one key element missing. Here-and-now work requires closeness and trust, the all-important *therapeutic alliance*. If that is lacking, offering difficult feedback is likely to feel uncomfortable or threatening. And I had not been able to build that bridge of trust with Alberto quickly, as I'd been focused so much on the struggle to communicate. Still, our time was running out, so I decided to take the plunge. It would either work or perhaps fail spectacularly, eliciting anger or resentment.

"Alberto, I want to reflect something back to you. I'm having a great deal of difficulty understanding what you're saying. At the beginning of our session I thought it was a technical problem with either Zoom or my hearing aids. After a bit I realized that my hearing was not the problem. The trouble lies, I believe, in the particular way you speak. You are trying hard to communicate with me but there is a kind of vagueness and over-complexity of your language that obscures your meaning and hinders my connection with you."

I glanced at my printout of Alberto's original message. "Consider these lines you sent, telling me that you wished to address 'the departing of veteran generations; views on the generation at hand; the possible (lack of) psychotherapy and psychoanalysis in the future.' Do you see how puzzling these phrases might seem to me? The problem is not with your English, which is excellent. And yet I'm trying very hard to follow you but failing." I paused before making my larger point. "And I suspect that my reaction mirrors how others must respond to you as well. I imagine they must often be perplexed by your words."

I really did not know what to expect. There was a good chance he would be offended and would attribute the problem to me: other English speakers have no problem understanding him—perhaps I was too old and slow to follow along.

Instead he seemed fascinated and responded immediately and nondefensively. "Irv, I appreciate your honesty. Know that you have company. Others, many others, have made similar comments to me. My girlfriend says the same thing. Over and over, she keeps telling me that I am too nebulous for her to follow, and that is when I'm speaking in Italian, our native language. You've put your finger exactly on what I wanted to discuss with you."

I was pleasantly surprised. But I knew the work was only halfway done, and there was no time to lose.

"Good. Alberto, your words are now very clear, and I understand why you contacted me. But let's look back at the email for a moment. Reading it again, there is no way in the world I would know that this is what you wished to examine. What a puzzle! On the one hand, you want to be close to others— you state this was the very reason you sought me out. But somehow you use your language as a way of keeping them at a distance. Does this resonate?"

"Go on, please," he said, staring fixedly at me.

"You want some help from me, but you conceal what help you seek. You want connection but make it impossible for others to connect. We are facing a mystery. Alberto, do you have any hunches about why you keep others at such a distance?"

"*Invasione*," he answered immediately.

"What?"

"*Invasione*. That's Italian for 'invasion.' *Invasione* sprung into my mind as soon as you asked why I keep others at a distance."

I was about to say something encouraging, like "Now we're talking!" but he didn't seem to need my applause and continued directly.

"And then *aggressione*. Italian for 'aggression.'"

"This sounds extremely important, Alberto. Please, try to focus on *aggressione* for a couple of minutes."

"I . . . hmm. I can't go any farther right now, but I can tell you with some certainty it has been a part of me all my life."

"Tell me, Alberto, are you experiencing *aggressione* with me today?" I'd expected a quick "no," but instead he sat pondering this question. Feeling the pressure of time ticking, I nudged a bit. "What does *aggressione* evoke for you? *Aggressione* from whom? *Aggressione* about what?"

Alberto shook his head. "Here's where my problem shows itself. I'm certain you want to help me, and I feel trust in you, but, even so, I feel a need arising to protect myself, to keep my distance. It's unclear . . . murky. I can't really express it right in English. Or maybe not in any language."

He was doing well, trying to open up here. I thought I'd gotten through to him and, as is often the case with these sessions, I began to suggest that it was the perfect time for him to enter ongoing therapy, when he cut me off abruptly.

"Therapy, therapy, yes okay, talk to someone every week about . . . what? . . . my childhood perhaps. But please tell me how might therapy help? What would I learn that might change *invasione* and *aggressione*?"

His defenses had sprung up already. Such powerful resistance. How could I address this in the few minutes we had left?

"Do you want anyone to know you deeply? To really know Alberto?" I asked.

"Very much so."

"I understand you have fears of being invaded or attacked. Perhaps some are appropriate. But because of these fears you only reveal a surface version of yourself, and an inscrutable one at that. No one gets to know the real you, and you never get to relax and just be yourself. It must be exhausting to maintain! And the end result is that you are not getting any deep intimacy, from Emma or anyone else."

"I see the problem," he said with a sigh. "And what would I do in therapy to address this?"

"I can't speak for every therapist, but I hope you would work together on becoming more comfortable with yourself. Your authentic self. Both internally, and eventually in how you relate to others. This might even mean being okay with showing the world some of your imperfections."

He kept nodding, a look of serious concentration on his face.

"I can imagine," I continued, "that bringing down your verbal defenses will let Emma feel closer to you. You might even end up enjoying yourself more."

"Those would be excellent results. I am intrigued, more than I expected."

"We've run out of time, but there's something I must say to you, something I've been experiencing. I am wondering who this person is I've been speaking with these last ten minutes. This is not the same Alberto I was speaking with during the first part of our session. This is not the same Alberto who so feared getting too close that he created a verbal fence around himself lest he face *invasione*. Did I pronounce it right?"

"You did quite well," he said, and then with a smile added, "for an American."

"I'm feeling much closer to you, Alberto. What has it been like for you?"

"This is a new experience for me, a rare experience. I imagine you probably encounter this often, this feeling of being *simpatico*. Pleasant, perhaps?"

"Yes, these last moments together have been very pleasant." I said nothing of the panic I'd felt earlier, imagining his convoluted verbosity to be an indicator of my own mental collapse. Not being able to fully trust my own capacities and perceptions was unsettling, and added a significant layer of challenge. As always, focusing on the patient right here, right now, helped ground me.

"You are at a wonderful transition, willing to examine yourself and take chances with new behavior. My hope is you'll experience such moments when you relate like this to your girlfriend and others whom you wish to know better. Do you know of any Italian therapists whom you could contact? If not, I can suggest some English-speaking ones who work via Zoom."

"I know one therapist in my city whom I respect very highly."

"Great. I urge you to contact them right away. Also, would you please send me an email in a few weeks. I would like an update on the powers of *aggressione* and *invasione*, and whether you're allowing Emma and others to sneak past the barricades."

In the previous couple of months I had taken to requesting some sort of follow-up from my patients, as I did here with Alberto. This was inspired by curiosity about two things. First, a great pleasure of being a therapist is that you are given a window into the compelling dramas of so many people's lives. I have often found myself caught up in these plots, wondering what happens next, cheering for my protagonist to thrive, a bit like watching an exciting television series. From this selfish perspective, the single consultation is an impoverished format and a follow-up email helps appease my curiosity a bit.

Far more important was a clinical curiosity about these consultations. I would never know the longer-term changes and growth these patients might experience, but I sorely wanted to know whether I was making any appreciable impact and, if so, which factors were most useful. Generally I'd been able to identify or clarify the patient's most pressing issue and found that most were concerned with their connection to others, which was no surprise to me. At heart, the huge majority of the patients I've seen over six decades are struggling in one way or another with interpersonal connection. Their immediate needs may present as something else—sexual obsession, anger at a parent, depression—but underneath these are often manifestations of disconnection. Even for those who present with extreme death anxiety, once we move below the surface, we nearly always find a longing for deep closeness with which to combat feelings of being alone in the universe. Clearly need for connection had been the case with Alberto.

What else could I glean? For one, that building the intimacy necessary for successful here-and-now work can be very challenging in such a short period of time. In my habitual therapy work I had built the trusting relationship with patients over weeks and months, and our capacity to do powerful work in the here and now grew with time. With Alberto, I had to rush ahead before that alliance was fully secure. I felt I'd been lucky with the positive way Alberto responded. In fact, I'd had a bit of luck with both Alberto and Maya of the forest puppy fantasy. In both cases I had taken a shortcut from my accustomed practice. With Maya I had been overly confrontational in asserting that her romantic relationship was at risk rather than helping her see that for herself. And with Alberto I had leapt to reflecting a difficult personal truth before we had established a clearly trusting relationship. Either case could easily have gone poorly, and yet my choices had seemed necessary in the shortened time horizon.

Looking back, I suspect the fact that both of them felt confidence in me before we met, given my stature in the field and sage gray-haired appearance, and had some sense of personal connection from reading my books had tilted the luck plane slightly in favor of positive outcomes. Clearly, establishing a warm, trusting relationship to the extent possible, as quickly as possible, was critical.

Trusting my intuition had also seemed important. Sometimes I had to take a leap based on no more than a feeling, as I had with Paul and the questions about his writing, which had worked out well. In the case of Christine, on the other hand, when I showed off by guessing that she had a troubled relationship to her father, things had gone less well—although here I believe the intuition had been on target, but my use of it was flawed. If the father relationship were critical, I should have teased it out over the course of the session rather than jumping to what was a bewildering conclusion for her. Intuition is highly important for therapists, but it's important to note that "intuition" as I view it is nothing mystical. Whatever intuition I have is the result of many decades of careful attention, of observing people closely, and recognizing patterns and tendencies.

I needed time to build enough trust to convey powerful messages in these single sessions—whether that was preparing someone for longer-term therapy, helping them see themselves in a new light, or modeling intimacy for them. Moving forward I would pay particular attention to the process of building trust and intimacy as quickly as I could. Hopefully my deteriorating brain would prove up to the task for a bit longer!

CHAPTER 9

Windows of Why, Whispers of When

H ana, a psychotherapist in Australia, sent me an enticing email that began:

> *I woke up this morning saying, "So many windows of why. So many whispers of when." I feel a lingering sense of sadness for a poem that wants to be written. I would love to explore these threads with you.*

Like most writers I am intrigued by unusual phrases, and Hana's "windows of why" and "whispers of when" enchanted me. I did not know exactly what she meant, or wanted to explore, but I was very curious to find out.

When we faced each other over Zoom a few days later in our session, she seemed timid, even frightened, and often stumbled over her words as she spoke through a cautious smile. Where was that poetic Hana who had written those otherworldly lines?

"I'm forty-nine years old, a mother of three children," she told me, in a rather halting way. "The older two are launched and live nearby with their partners. My youngest is seventeen and has just graduated from high school. He will start college as soon as COVID permits. As for me, I live and work in Melbourne as a therapist. I guess I have an existential bent—you've been a major influence, and I know your books and theories well. I'm in private practice, and all my patients are on Zoom now, of course. I do miss the in-person contact. Me and most everyone else on the planet! What else should you know? My mother and my three sisters live in New Zealand, and I was about to visit them when the travel restrictions descended."

She paused, then gave a quick nod to indicate she'd finished. That seemed a quick, concise rundown of a lot of identifying information, but nothing pressing.

"What issues are troubling you now?" I asked.

"Hmmm. First, my therapist of ten years has recently retired. Second, I am anxious about my son leaving home," she said. "Also, I am having issues with my husband. We've been married twenty-five years, but we're just hanging on by a thread right now."

I waited for her to continue but she said nothing more. After a short silence I prodded her. "Your marriage is hanging by a thread. That sounds important, Hana. And you save that for last because . . . ?"

"Because I am an eternal optimist and believe in hope and healing."

I noted that she deflected my question and guessed that her marriage must be a source of pain. I took care to be gentle. "Hana, I'm guessing that it's not easy for you to speak about your marriage, but I imagine you'd be very disappointed if we didn't address it."

"Yes, yes, my marriage. I need to get into couples therapy. I have a therapist in mind, but my husband won't give me an answer. I'm still patiently waiting for him to make up his mind."

I remained silent, expecting more, but she simply maintained a cautious smile. She fidgeted a bit and adjusted her screen but did not continue speaking. *That's it?* I thought. *That's all she is going to say?* Several minutes passed, and I wondered whether I should comment on our process. *Why does she offer me so little? Why does she keep forcing me to ask her questions?* I chose not to comment yet on our here-and-now relationship, what was going on between us in the conversation, and particularly my sense that she was being somehow evasive. I thought there must be some key information that I hadn't gotten yet and that much would become clear when I did. "Please tell me more about your relationship with your husband," I said.

"The marriage is simply not working. I really don't know why."

Simply not working! Once again, precious little information. And why did she keep saying "the marriage" rather than "my marriage" or "our marriage"? How odd. She knew she needed help and that we only had one short hour to talk. I thought she'd be eager to offer more information that would help us get to the heart of the matter. Instead, though the minutes were ticking rapidly by, she volunteered the stingiest glimpses, waiting for me to pose questions, which she invariably deflected. I felt my patience beginning to erode. After all, she was a therapist who undoubtedly knew the importance of opening up and sharing herself and her deep concerns. And as I was learning, if I were to be helpful, it was crucial to move very quickly.

I pushed a little harder.

"Your hunches, Hana, about *why* your marriage is not working?"

"Well, I've wanted us to get into some couples therapy. I

found a good therapist who can see us, but so far my husband won't respond to my suggestion."

She'd already said this. How could I get past the resistance?

"Hana, can you give me more details about your relationship with your husband? I have little idea of what's happening between the two of you. How long has the marriage been hanging by a thread?"

"Oh, a while now. A couple of years."

"And what's the sleeping arrangement? And your sexual life?"

"He snores so much that we've slept in different bedrooms for many years. There hasn't been sex for ages."

"Are you two intimate in other ways? Close, caring?"

"Not really."

Such short, stingy answers. I suspected she contributed to the problems with her husband by talking to him in the same terse, deflecting manner. But why respond to me like this, now? She knew my therapeutic approach emphasized the relationship between us in the here and now, and yet she continued to avoid connecting. Without a stronger sense of trust I was wary of looking critically at what was going on between us, and so I again took another tack.

"Hana, what options do you have if your husband continues not to answer your invitation to start couples therapy?"

"I've got a few," Hana replied. "The most extreme is to return to my roots in New Zealand where my mother and my sisters live. Before we got married I had a nice psychotherapy practice there, and I'm confident I can rebuild it. I'm really considering this."

"Hana," I said, "I am quite concerned that sometime in the future when you review your life you're going to experience profound regret for not confronting whatever is going on in your marriage, for not attempting to change things."

She waited calmly as I spoke, then said, "I do have a local individual therapist in mind, and I plan to schedule a meeting with her. I also plan to confront my husband about his procrastination."

I glanced at my watch and was stunned to see our time was up. Hana and I said a genial goodbye, after a session that felt to me as if we were, not just in body but in spirit, continents away from each other.

I felt dismayed that I had offered her so little. Why hadn't I focused on our here-and-now relationship the way I always do? And what had happened to the time? It had raced by. I felt discouraged. I should have been able to offer her more yet was unsure about what I could have done. This was surely one of my least successful consultations.

That night, when I was attempting and failing to sleep, I again found myself thinking about my session with Hana. I was flooded with the questions I had not posed: *Why don't you talk to your husband about your relationship? Why just suggest couples therapy instead of insisting upon it? Does your husband know how unhappy you are with the relationship? That you're thinking of leaving him, not to mention leaving the country? And why don't you insist on more from your marriage? Where did you learn never to complain or that you have no right to ask for anything?*

I had other unasked questions about my role and our relationship in our session. *Why did you make me work so hard? You're an experienced therapist, and you know my approach well, so why did I have to make such effort to find out what's troubling you?*

The therapist in me felt discouraged by my ineptitude. At the same time, for reasons I could not completely explain, the teaching writer in me told me there was an interesting story in here somewhere, even if I didn't know what it was yet. The next morning, I decided to contact Hana about exploring our hour together in writing. I generally do this after I have finished a story, but Hana, and whatever had happened in our session, was such an enigma that I did not want to invest a great deal of time writing about our session, only to have her turn me down. I sent her this email:

Hi Hana,

Since our consultation, I've been thinking of writing a short story about our meeting. I'm not clear what the finished product would say, but it would mostly examine my own feelings during our session and my not entirely successful attempt to grasp what you are going through.

Rest assured, I always go to great lengths to disguise patients' identity in every possible way so that no one on earth would recognize the protagonist. I'm eager to start but I don't want to begin writing if you have any objections.

Thank you, Irv

Given how unhelpful I'd been during the session, I placed the odds of her saying "yes" at about 4 to 1 against. But several hours later Hana greatly surprised me:

Dear Irv,

Today is my birthday. Your email requesting to write this story is maybe the best gift I've received in my life! I am both honored and terrified.

You have long been my answer to the question, "Who is one person, dead or alive, that you'd like to spend an hour with?" How does it feel to be on someone's bucket list?

Since our consultation I have felt cracked wide open. It

feels uncomfortable in just the way it should. I thought I had no expectations for an outcome when we met, but I am aware now that I hoped to come away with a sense of elation. What I did not expect was to feel so raw, and so angry with you! How dare you continue to probe? And now here you are, revisiting the probing!

But you are the master of trusting your instincts. Your books have given me permission to use myself as the instrument of my work, and to trust that the relationship is where the healing occurs. Last night after our powerful meeting, I began to wonder what it was like for you after we hung up. I was having a life-shifting experience. And you? Just carrying on, after notching session number 789,397,986 on your belt?

Please feel free to write the story. I am eager to read it!

With respect and adoration,

Hana

I responded immediately:

I loved your letter, Hana. Wow, you're already a very, very different Hana. This Hana is not going to be silent with her husband about working on their relationship. This Hana is not timid. She will demand an answer. This is the Hana who wrote of "windows of why and whispers of when."

Please don't be uneasy about the story. Anything I write will be benign as far as our relationship goes! Thank you for the go-ahead, and I will send you a draft if I can manage to write it.

Happy birthday, Irv

The following day I received a very illuminating email from Hana:

I've been thinking nonstop of you trying to write our story, continually slamming up against unanswered questions, perhaps wanting to quit. I could see your frustration during our session. No doubt you felt you had to work too hard. You must have been baffled by my evading so many of your inquiries. You must have wondered why I offered so little of myself.

I am feeling so much compassion for you that I've now decided to come to your rescue! You are puzzled about our session because you're overlooking something crucial. Something so very, very obvious: you are my model, my teacher. You changed my life. I decided to become a therapist because of your books. I have read every one of them, and their pages are dog-eared and covered with notes. Here's what you overlooked, the missing link. I want your approval and your love! Above all, I want you to admire me. But there are things, some dark shameful things about me, particularly about my behavior in my marriage, that I cannot, will not, reveal to you. Hence my reticence.

Now, armed with this information, please go ahead and write our story!

Hana

Her response startled me. The pieces began to fall into place, why I'd been able to get so little out of her during our session, why my approach had been so ineffective. I had been blind to the great reverence in which she held me and hadn't noticed this affecting our therapy. As previously noted, I have often been able to leverage the admiration with which patients hold me, using it to speed up the process or to give my thoughts and pronouncements added weight in their minds. *If the esteemed Dr. Irvin Yalom gives approval, I must be doing something right!* Or *If Dr. Irvin Yalom advises X, I should immediately do it.*

With Hana, however, my being *Dr. Irvin Yalom* backfired! Worse, I didn't notice this was happening during our session and kept drilling away at the one area, her marriage, where she felt most vulnerable. I have long believed that therapists are most effective when we offer ourselves to our patients as fellow travelers, human beings who must also suffer the slings and arrows and other indignities of being alive. This differs sharply with the positioning of many in the field historically, and even now, who present themselves as experts, there to *fix* their patients, as if the human condition were fixable. Perhaps by relying too heavily on my status in these single sessions, I had inadvertently slid too far in that direction.

Deep down I know that honest sharing about myself as a normal, flawed, mortal human being—one besieged by my own doubts and anxieties—is both normalizing of the patient's troubles and a catalyst for the intimacy and trust needed for change. My humanity and personhood are critical, and with Hana I had not offered enough of them. Encountering my public persona (laden with such esteem and admiration) may indeed be useful for some, but it can also have the opposite effect, shutting people like Hana down.

Why hadn't I noticed this during the session? Likely I'd become overconfident in my influence. To answer Hana's question, being on someone's bucket list is a bit intoxicating. But I know it is much better as a therapist not to emphasize one's position of acclaim but rather to get down in the mud with one's patients and slog together through our absurd and challenging world. I'll have to be aware of how intimidating being *Dr. Irvin Yalom* may be in the future, particularly when working with other therapists. There may be moments when using the amplified importance of my persona is helpful, but in general I'll attempt simply to be Irv.

CHAPTER 10

Alone, Alone, Alone

Margaret's brief email informed me that she was a sixty-five-year-old math teacher living in Melbourne, Australia, who suffered from great loneliness and frequent panic attacks. She wrote that since the beginning of the pandemic she had been waking at night from frightening dreams that left her gasping and wishing for help. Alas, she was alone, very alone.

"I was diagnosed with autism when I was fourteen. So I have my limitations," she concluded.

Two weeks later I opened a Zoom window and encountered an intense, silver-haired woman whose lips twitched with anxiety.

"Let's start right in, Margaret. From your email I know that you're lonely and often nervous. Please tell me more about yourself."

"I hardly know how to start. I'm not good at talking. Talking to anyone. I never have been. I spend almost all my time alone."

"Tell me more about that. Loneliness is quite common right

now, with all of us in our COVID bubbles. It is a very strange time."

"For me, it's different. I've been alone my entire life. Alone since day one."

"Please, you lead."

She gave me a quick, bleak review of her life. When she said she had been alone since day one, she meant it literally, as her mother had died in childbirth. Then, when Margaret was five, her father had deserted the family, never to be heard from again. She and her brother, who was seven years older, had been raised by her maternal grandmother, an elderly woman who kept a stern, quiet household.

As Margaret went on I was stunned by her degree of isolation, first in childhood and then through adolescence into a lonely adulthood. At no point did she mention a friend or any important relationships. As she spoke, desolate images appeared unbidden in my mind: empty hallways, deserted school rooms in summertime, beach resorts in gray winter light.

I probed further, hoping I would discover someone who cared for her.

"Who are you closest to now, Margaret?" I asked. This question almost always opens doors in therapy, nudging people to think beyond themselves and to focus on the wider web of relationships in which they live. But she spoke of only one important person in her life—her brother, a French teacher. He was also unmarried, and lived in another city several hundred miles away. They had not been together in person for over a decade, but they spoke on the phone regularly for exactly ten minutes, once each week.

"Why exactly ten minutes?"

"Ten minutes is correct," she said.

"No more, no less?"

"Correct."

"And why?"

She gestured with her hand, as if to say that this was some-how preordained, a limitation not to be questioned. Then she went on to tell me she had supported herself as a mathematics teacher until her retirement a year ago. She had always lived alone. She listened to her collection of classical music albums and spent hours carefully preparing her meals. Here I noted a brief smile appear on her face, as she described in some detail the meticulous cooking and laying out of precise menus, the specifics of the food clearly important to her.

I asked her when she had last shared a meal with another person. She could not remember; perhaps several years ago. As she related the details of her past and current life I felt quite uneasy. Margaret began to cry, copious tears pouring freely as she described a life empty of all significant relationships. Her loneliness was so extreme that I was shaken somewhat from my habitual position in which I felt deeply for patients' suffering but generally managed to keep myself calm enough to re-main helpful. Now I could feel myself becoming unsettled, the echoes of my own terribly lonely childhood rippling just below the surface. I wanted badly to soothe her, while also keeping my own discomfort in check, but no useful interventions came to mind—no insightful reframing of her situation, no clever shift of perspective to ameliorate her sense of self. All I could manage were sympathetic utterances of support, *Mmm, that's very hard* and *I can only imagine your fear.*

Then she told me that she had recently submitted an essay for an anthology about the experiences of children who grew up feeling different from other children, but she had never even received a response. Here was a possible point of connection!

"Ouch, I know how much that must hurt, Margaret. Being

a fellow writer, and one who has received a fair share of rejections, I can appreciate your pain."

After a brief silence, she took a deep breath, and said, "My essay is short, one thousand three hundred words. Approximately. I doubt if anyone else in the world will ever read it. I . . . I . . . wonder if I could read it aloud to you."

"Of course. I'd like very much to hear it."

She broke into a true smile and then began reading. It was a well-written, heart-wrenching essay about her sense of estrangement in grade school and her many failed attempts to make friends with other children. I made a point of listening intently and taking a few notes. This took about fifteen minutes, longer than I expected, but I could sense her pleasure at my attentiveness.

When she finished, I commented that, as a fellow writer, I admired her excellent prose, and I asked her to read again several of the sentences that particularly moved me. I pointed out that she and I shared several things: "You and I are dedicated readers, we adore fine literature, and we both take great pleasure in crafting a robust sentence."

She said something that I had trouble hearing, but which I believe was "thank you for listening." She was smiling and looked directly at the camera. For a brief instant we were connected, present together in the resonance of her prose. A lovely moment. Then a flash of hesitation crossed her face, and she glanced down. I could feel the closeness collapsing, distance pouring in. I needed to hold on to that connection before the space between yawned open, and I reached across, saying, "Margaret, there's something else I want to tell you. I'm really attuned to your loneliness right now. It's not only the pandemic, although that has cloistered me in my home. It's an even deeper isolation stemming from my wife's death a few

112   •   HOUR OF THE HEART

months ago. She and I met each other when we were fourteen, so I've never really been alone as an adult. I had a terribly solitary childhood, and I've always thought of her as having saved me. Right now, I think I can identify with your isolation. Really I suspect you have much to teach me."

I hadn't thought to share this very personal information until the moment I did so. Marilyn's death had entered several recent consultations, but always brought up by patients who had read her obituary in some newspaper or magazine and wanted to offer me their condolences. This was the first time I had revealed it myself, and I had a flash of second-guessing. But it seemed potentially useful for Margaret to hear, an offer of my own vulnerability in a gambit to bring us closer.

She was clearly taken aback, confused by my revelation. She hesitated for a few moments, then opened her mouth to speak but could utter no words. Finally, she said, "Sorry, so sorry . . ." then continued, "My brother calls, but we don't talk about much. I think he—"

"Margaret, let me ask you something." I sensed her moving away and interrupted, bringing our focus to the here and now. "How did you feel just now when I told you about my losing my wife? What was that like for you?"

"Uh, uh, no one has ever said anything like that to me, something so, so . . . I don't know . . . so personal. Connection. And then . . . I couldn't answer you . . . I didn't know what to say."

"Try to recall what passed through your mind as you thought about what to say."

"Uh, uh, fear. For the most part, fear. I felt something was expected of me—something I wasn't up to. You even said that *you* could learn from *me*."

"Yes. And?"

"I felt . . . um . . . empty. After all, I am autistic. What do I have to offer you?"

"Margaret, you're far too hard on yourself. I'm so sorry that we're coming to the end of our time together, but before we stop I have one important question. What are your feelings about how you and I are doing in our meeting today?"

Margaret looked at me a bit quizzically.

"Tell me," I said. "Do you think the two of us have had an intimate encounter?"

She nodded vigorously. "Absolutely."

"And is this intimacy good?"

"Yes. Oh yes."

"I agree entirely, Margaret. I feel the same way. I feel it keenly."

"Thank you."

"Ah. I should thank *you*, Margaret. It takes *two* to create such an encounter."

She suddenly began weeping loudly. I let the tears run for a moment, then said, "I'm so moved by your reaction. It's important to experience and express your feelings. You're far more capable of it than you think."

"Autistic people don't relate."

"I can't speak about autistic people. But I just experienced Margaret relating, and I believe you're selling yourself short."

She continued weeping.

"I am afraid I will always be alone."

"In my field, Margaret, we refer to that idea as a 'self-fulfilling prophecy.' In other words, you play a role in what happens to your relationships. If I had to choose one thing from our hour today that I hope you'll remember, it is this: *you and I had a real encounter.* Right?"

She nodded her head vigorously as she wiped her tears away.

"And, Margaret, *it takes two to create an encounter. You did this with me.*"

At the end of the session, I suggested that she look into local support groups for people on the spectrum. I also thought she would benefit from individual therapy and gave her the information for a fine therapist I knew in Melbourne.

A few weeks later I reached out to this colleague and learned that he had not heard from Margaret. I was concerned and emailed Margaret suggesting, once again, that she contact the therapist.

A day later Margaret sent a long email saying that she didn't feel she needed to pursue therapy just then. Her closing words:

I was particularly touched by your response to my writing. Your listening and liking my essay meant a lot. And after our talk I felt that I am not in such a bad place. I got what I wanted for our session. In fact, I got more: a greater sense of self-worth and confidence. For now, that is enough for me.

Thank you.

I thought about Margaret a great deal in the weeks that followed. Her extreme loneliness haunted me, and perhaps also served as a reality check for my own self-pity when I felt most alone. Even without Marilyn, and in the midst of COVID, I had my children who visited, my daily sessions with patients, and a wonderful young man, Joe, who had recently moved into my house to help care for me. Perhaps *I* was not in such a bad place. I knew I could not stand the tremendous isolation in which Margaret lived, but I suspect the kinds and degrees of connection we all want are quite different from each other. If meeting with me once felt like enough connection for Margaret right now, who was I to disagree?

I sometimes imagined her working with a therapist and what that might be like. And I imagined her connecting with others in real life, perhaps meeting through a support group, perhaps through a chance encounter in the classical music section of a local record store. Eventually I wrote this story and sent it to her for permission to publish. I did not hear back. I had completely given up the idea of including it in this book when, two years later, a surprising email appeared. She gave permission for the story to be published but asked that this coda be included:

> *Since my single-session encounter with Dr Yalom, my life and lifestyle have changed considerably. In 2022, after more than three decades, I returned to the Christian faith that I adopted when I was 19 years old.*
>
> *This means I have accepted Christ as the Jewish Messiah and as Lord and Saviour; '. . . but one thing I do, forgetting those things which are behind and reaching forward to those things which are ahead,' Philippians 3:13.*

I will never know exactly how things have shifted for Margaret, but now I imagine her connecting with someone at a church event. I am far from religious, but I do appreciate many of the things religion has to offer, particularly community and acceptance, which would be so good for her.

CHAPTER 11

Bartering

I hadn't planned to speak to Margaret about Marilyn's death and my loneliness. It had simply happened in the course of our conversation, when I felt her slipping further away from me and had reached out for connection. The effects were powerful. It had immediately created a shift in our relationship such that a deeply intimate moment was possible between myself and Margaret, for whom sharing of self was fraught with anxiety. This had led to emotional release and a profound experience for both of us.

This sharing from my own life story is an example of *self-disclosure*, that is, a therapist offering information about themselves to their patients with the intention of advancing the therapy. By and large most people envision therapists as being question askers, listeners, occasional prodders, and cheerleaders. Depending on one's particular theoretical approach, we might also expect them to be educators, assigners of homework, and prescribers of medication. But we don't often think of them as talking too much about themselves.

At its core, therapy is an unusual and, in many ways, one-sided relationship: the patient engages in a great deal of self-reflection and revelation, while the therapist focuses intensely on the patient and reveals very little of themselves.

There are many reasons why therapists are trained not to bring their own stories and personal information into therapy. Historically, psychiatry grew out of a medical model, in which the doctor was positioned as the expert, the patient as "ill" and in need of curing. Psychiatrists projected the high status of Physician, and what problems were uncovered were seen entirely as faults or flaws that the good doctor could repair. Additionally, Freud's original psychoanalytic model had, embedded in it, the dynamic of the therapist as a blank screen onto which patients would project their feelings, fantasies, and neuroses. Too much information about the therapist as a human being would taint this dynamic, influencing the patient's process of self-discovery.

I will note here that well over a hundred years have passed since Freud's revolutionary work, and countless other brilliant thinkers and practitioners have made contemporary therapy rich and varied, with many approaches that differ widely from this blank screen approach. Nonetheless, remnants of the aloof, expert doctor ideal persists, and most training programs continue to caution against therapists sharing deeply of themselves.

Most of the reasons for such a stance have always seemed rather poor to me, and I have long been very far on the "reveal more" side of the field when it comes to this question. Being a fellow traveler rather than a distant expert has been one of my guiding principles for decades. One type of self-disclosure is absolutely central to my here-and-now work: being deeply honest as to how I feel about a patient in the immediate present.

I don't blurt out my feelings indiscriminately, of course, but rather use these as my main source of data and carefully consider how I can best employ this information to the patient's benefit. For example, if a patient appears to be withholding something, I ask about that; if they are being combative, or flirtatious, or childish, I let them know in the most useful way I can that this is what I am receiving from them.

A second type of self-disclosure is relating personal experiences or stories from my life in the service of the patient's therapy. This is really the self-disclosure that most young therapists are cautioned to avoid, as if there is some great danger here—perhaps that the therapist appearing as a normal, flawed human being will somehow lessen our curative capacity, or perhaps that being honest about one's life is somehow too taxing for therapists. And yet patients will often ask direct questions about their therapists, from whether we have children to what our political views are. Should we ignore them? One common tactic that therapists employ when a patient does so is to flip the question around and wonder why the patient is interested in knowing these things. It is true that sometimes a patient's questions can be revealing of something deeper in their personality. For instance, a patient who asks constantly how a therapist is doing may be revealing their own tendency to adopt a caretaker role in their relationships while simultaneously shifting focus away from their own problems. But most of the time I believe patients ask such questions simply because they want to know more about the person with whom they are building an important relationship. They want to know who we are, to see if we have enough in common to understand their challenges or to calm their anxiety about this strange, structured relationship. What's the big deal here?

If a patient wants to know what kind of television shows I like, I'm happy to tell them. Do I have children? How do I feel about a certain restaurant? How did I get along with my parents? Why should I hide such things? How can I nurture the true human connection so essential to helping patients if I am afraid to share myself?

Possibly there is concern that too much intimacy may lead to a blurring of roles and that the closeness of therapy may inspire romantic feelings on the part of either patient or therapist. This is certainly possible—after all, for many the therapist is the person they share with most deeply. And it is certainly a problem if ever it does arise. Yet I firmly believe that we trained professional therapists can be careful enough and self-aware enough to avoid this, and to examine such romantic or sexual feelings appropriately if they do arise.

What is critical, of course, is that our sharing be in the best interest of the patient. And there may well be circumstances where too much sharing, or sharing certain things, is detrimental. But, and let me emphasize this point, in my six-plus decades of doing therapy, I don't believe I have had the experience of sharing too much with a negative impact. On the contrary, my self-disclosure always seems to bring me and my patients closer together and to improve the course of therapy.

With Margaret and several other recent patients, facts about my own life had entered into our conversations, including Marilyn's death and some memories from my childhood. While these personal experiences may not, at first glance, appear directly relevant to patients' presenting problems, my offering them ended up being beneficial. How? I suspect that it accelerated the pace of developing trust and intimacy between us, helping the patients become comfortable enough to open up about their own experiences more rapidly. This was a key realization in single-session work, as the major difference between this and my accustomed longer-term therapy was, of course, the sense of urgency. No longer could I wait weeks to build a powerful relationship with the patient before going deeper into issues. Rather, I had to move quickly to build connection, and I was learning that this was an excellent tool.

So far these bits of self-disclosure had been mostly unplanned, instigated by a patient's kind concern about my grief or, as with Margaret, my spontaneous gambit at connection. I decided that the next time I had an appropriate opportunity with a patient who felt distant or evasive, I would intentionally experiment with bringing in more of myself more quickly, even if it felt rushed or premature compared to how I have done so in the past.

I only had to wait a few days. One morning in September 2020, Beatriz's striking face with dark Mediterranean features appeared on my computer screen. She was in Portugal and, speaking clear English, she launched into our session: "I am thirty-three, married for eleven years, and have a four-year-old daughter. I am a painter, and here is my current work." She stepped to the side, revealing a large unfinished painting of two small boats sailing into a fiery setting sun. It was beautiful. "This is the Atlantic, seen from my studio on the third floor of my home," she added.

"What a gorgeous painting!" I said. "And how fortunate you are to have such a view."

"Dr. Yalom—"

"Call me Irv, please."

"Irv, then. I'm so glad you like my painting." She drew a quick breath. "Can I be spontaneous? A thought just sailed into my mind. I'm wondering if you'd be interested in bartering this painting for your fee for our session?"

This was a first! At my age, it's a kick to run into something entirely new. I had a hunch this hour was going to be quite a ride.

I tried to respond in a cordial manner. "Over a great many years of practice, Beatriz, I've learned that it's always best to keep the therapy and the fee quite—um—separate."

I felt like a horribly uptight prude, but what else could I say? She reacted with a playful smile. She was really enjoying this. Good for her. For a moment I considered suggesting we look at this interchange in depth. But it was too early to examine our process. We had just begun.

"So," I said, "let's get right to work, Beatriz. Your email was brief, and I know very little about you. Tell me the issues you'd like to work on in our session. What's happening in your life now that prompted you to contact me?"

"What's happening? Quite a bit. My father has been traveling with his buddies so my sister and I have had to spend a lot of time with my mother. All of those relationships are more or less fine, but it's a lot of hours with family. Let's see. Another thing is that I am an aficionado of psychology literature. I read on the topic constantly, from theory to new studies. I read several of your books recently and loved them. So I thought I might get a lot from speaking with you. Those are some answers."

"And how do you think I can be of help?"

"I guess the *real* reason I'm contacting you is my relationship with my husband, João. He is a biologist, and extremely smart. For the last six months he has been a high-level researcher for a company trying to develop a COVID vaccine. He has always worked hard. But now, it's really too much. Over and over, he keeps reminding me that it is *important work*. He makes good money, more than he's ever made, but his hours are insane: he comes home near midnight every night. Some days he'll come home for a short dinner and then rush back to work."

"Weekends?"

"The same."

"That doesn't leave much time for you and him to be close."

"I'm taking it that *close* means sex?"

"Could be. Whatever closeness you want with him."

"Well, our sex life is moribund."

"Moribund! Your English vocabulary is excellent."

"Three years in British boarding school and two years at Boston University." She smiled. "My English is certainly more excellent than our moribund sex life."

"Tell me—*how* moribund?"

"Several weeks can pass by."

"And is this new?"

"We used to be far more, how shall I say, frisky?"

We sat for a moment, her warm, playful demeanor resonant between us, but counterbalanced by obvious frustration. I tried to imagine what it was like for her, to have her husband be so distant.

"You say that he's working on finding a vaccine for corona-virus. That is indeed *important work*. Extremely important. It must be hard for you to complain to him about his working hours."

"As you Americans might say, '*Bingo!*'"

"Beatriz, let me tell you what I'm feeling. I don't know the ins and outs of the race for the COVID vaccine, but I imagine it's intensely high-pressured. Nevertheless, working till midnight seven days a week seems . . . unreal. I suspect he's working longer hours than any scientist in the world."

Beatriz chuckled.

I raised my eyebrows.

"It's funny because those were my exact words last week, just before he strode out of the house and slammed the door. Hard."

"This pace can't be good for his health, and it is clearly a disaster at home," I said. "You haven't mentioned it, but I can imagine this is hard for your daughter, too."

"She was upset at first, with COVID shutting her school, and then her father disappearing. By now she's almost forgotten who he is."

I felt perplexed. I wondered if *all* of this time were spent in the lab. It struck me that it could also be the cover for something clandestine that he did not want to share with Beatriz. Perhaps he was having an affair. Leaping to this suspicion was, admittedly, a big jump based on little information. But when there are such large behavioral shifts in a marriage and one partner simply can't understand why, infidelity is often involved. I felt certain there was something missing in the story Beatriz was presenting. Could it be another woman?

Beatriz was so warm and spirited that it was difficult for me to entertain the idea. She spoke playfully, as if whatever challenges she and her husband were having were part of a game, whereas I imagine discovering such an affair would be a serious rupture. I felt I had to explore the possibility, but I did not want to accidentally create a greater rift by implanting a suspicion if this were not the case, so I ventured very carefully. "Beatriz, I think there's some important missing piece to this mystery."

"I agree!" she said, almost conspiratorially. "But I don't know what it is. Do you have an idea?"

How to proceed with maximum caution? I tried to open the door gently. Affairs are usually a response to something amiss in the marriage, so I began there.

"I can't help wondering if there's something happening in your relationship that might be the *cause* of your husband's absence from home rather than the *result* of his absence."

"What? I'm not sure what you're saying."

"Whatever is going on in a marriage, it is the outcome of both people's contributions."

"What do you mean?"

She hadn't taken the bait. Again, I knew I needed to proceed with caution. A therapist can really only work with the person in the room, and there are limitations to how useful it is to speculate about the actions and motivation of others, so I chose once more not to ask directly if he might be having an affair. I continued to focus on her role.

"Do you think there might be things you've done to alienate him? To make him feel uncomfortable or uncared for?"

"I can't imagine," she said after the briefest reflection.

"Might he want more attention?"

"But I'm right here! He's the one who is never home."

Perhaps I wasn't being direct enough. Or perhaps she was willfully evading my implications.

"So as far as you know, you aren't doing anything that might make him feel more appreciated elsewhere?"

She looked dumbfounded, as if she'd just lost her English completely or I'd started speaking Hungarian. Aware that my suspicion was based on very little information, I decided to back off rather than express the idea of an affair openly. I could always return to it if needed.

"Okay. Let me ask, what happens when you and he talk about your relationship, about these feelings of distance?"

"We haven't. Not really."

"I don't know what is going on exactly, Beatriz, but I feel something serious is happening in your marriage. I urge you, strongly, to see a couples therapist who can help the two of you sort this out together and find your way back to each other."

Beatriz was silent.

"What do you feel when I say this?"

"Mixed feelings. Part of me knows you're right, but it feels unrealistic."

"How so?"

"My husband has *always* had negative feelings about therapy. He disputes this, but I think it goes back to his parents seeing a therapist and subsequently divorcing. He gets annoyed just noticing the books I read."

"And you don't think he could overcome that annoyance?"

"I doubt that he'd be willing," she said with some finality.

I felt stuck. It seemed clear that any real progress would require them both to be in the room together, working on their relationship. I'd suggested this very clearly, and she'd rejected it out of hand. What else could I do? Then, thinking about Beatriz and her husband, he so driven, she feeling abandoned and bewildered, a decades-old scene from my own marriage drifted into mind. Remembering my plan to experiment with self-disclosure, I decided to share it. Our time was ticking, and Beatriz seemed unwilling to dig deeper. Perhaps this might help.

"I'm reminded of a period in my own life, decades ago now," I began. "When I was first hired at Stanford, my wife, Marilyn, applied to be a professor of comparative literature—she was a brilliant scholar, and absolutely qualified for the position. Instead of being taken seriously, she was dismissed with the comment 'we don't hire faculty wives.' Well, after a decade of teaching undergraduate French at a much less prestigious university, Stanford *did* hire her, not as a professor but as one of the directors of its newly formed Center for Research on Women. We celebrated this victory.

"But soon she was deeply engaged and focused entirely on her new work, much like your husband. And after a few months, I remember feeling something like you might feel right now, entirely ignored by my spouse. I tried to be patient, sensing it wasn't fair for me to complain, given how fulfilled she clearly felt. When it got bad enough, I tried to bring it up with her several times, but she was too wrapped up in work to pay much attention. For the very first time, I felt dissatisfied with my marriage."

I hadn't thought about this period in years. Marilyn's face then came so clearly to me, her excitement as she embarked on a career involved with women's history and liberation. She was in her early forties, just a few years older than Beatriz. I was momentarily overcome with feelings—love, pleasure at the memory of our life together back then, when Palo Alto was still partially apricot orchards, and we were young enough to be embarking on new adventures. I believe I must have closed my eyes, because I opened them to see Beatriz's face and pulled myself back to the present moment. I couldn't get lost in my stories if they were going to be helpful to her.

"One evening," I continued, "we were having dinner at a restaurant in San Francisco. I was particularly frustrated with things as they stood, and I took the plunge. I told her I was pleased that her new job was so exciting but that she had become so preoccupied that our marriage was no longer working for me. I remember saying, 'I'm beginning to wonder if we should stay together . . .' at which point she began to wail. Very loudly. So loudly that everyone in the restaurant stopped eating and turned to stare at us. It was a shocking sound. I gestured to the waiter for the bill, paid it quickly, and we left the restaurant, Marilyn still sobbing. We walked toward our apartment and, after a couple of blocks, she reached out for my hand. We walked in silence, holding hands like we did in high school, and soon we were hugging each other as we had hugged when we were teenagers."

Beatriz's eyes were fixed on me as I wrapped up this old memory. There was a palpable shift between us, her face grown softer and less playful. After a moment, she spoke.

"Thank you for sharing. I'm not sure how to . . . well, just, thank you."

"If we were in ongoing therapy," I said, "I would want to focus on your powerlessness, the feeling that, because your husband is doing such important work, you have no right to question anything he does. I certainly felt something like that."

She nodded, still right there with me. My story had brought us close together, and it felt right to move into the here and now. The central mystery of why the marriage had grown distant remained, and perhaps examining what was happening between us would provide a clue, as it so often did.

"But our time is limited, Beatriz. So I'd like to make a different suggestion. Can we talk about our relationship? How are you and I doing in this session?"

She looked baffled.

"Confused? Let me put it this way: Can you give voice to the feelings you've had about me or about us in this past hour?"

"Uh . . . I don't know. I'm stuck. Help me out."

"Perhaps in your reading you've come across the idea of *free association*?"

"Yes . . . in Freudian analysis. The patient says everything that comes to mind."

"Exactly. I find this often helps get thoughts flowing when someone gets stuck, as you say. Can you try to free associate right now? Try to think out loud about our meeting today and what we've been talking about."

"I've never done this before."

"Try to let your mind go free."

"For how long?"

"Just a few minutes."

"I'll try," she said, closing her eyes. "I was very excited about our call. Wanted to tell you everything right away. But for some reason I . . . I started with that business about my painting . . . insisted on showing it to you . . . telling you that it was the view from my studio. Actually, I'm embarrassed about that."

"Why embarrassed?" I nudged.

"Wanted to show you what a good artist I am . . . wanted to have your attention and respect. And my offer of trading the painting for the hour of consultation—that was embarrassing— a bit crazy. But your response was a bit pompous, Dr. Yalom."

Beatriz paused, then opened her eyes with a quick laugh. "Well, maybe *pompous* was the wrong word. Your response to my offer felt like a put-down."

"Can you give voice to the feelings you have right now?"

"Well, it's complicated. I felt put down, almost scolded by you, and yet, at the same time, I was very much relieved. Frankly, I don't know what I would have done if you had accepted my offer of the painting for our hour. I'm a successful artist. It will take me many, many hours to finish the painting and my price for it would be more, many times more, than the fee for our consultation. So, thank you for saying no."

"Can you say more about *why* you made that offer?"

"Being playful. Perhaps flirtatious."

"That's it? I'm skeptical. Can you go deeper?"

"My goodness, Dr. Yalom, you are a persistent man! None of your writings point that out. *Deeper*, you ask. Well, perhaps I wanted you to know how talented I am. How important. Perhaps I wanted you to take me more seriously." Beatriz paused to think a minute. "Yes, I confess, I knew that a discussion of my offer would, in some way, lead to my telling you what my paintings really cost. The truth is that my paintings have supported us in a lavish manner. My husband and I started out with nothing. He was the one with a traditional career, and he was successfully climbing the ladder as an academic scientist. I don't think he took my artistic aspirations very seriously, and sometimes I didn't, either. Then I was noticed by a major gallery, and suddenly my paintings were selling for large sums of money. A successful solo show allowed us to buy this gorgeous house, with views of the sunset on one side and green hills of a national park on the other."

Ah! Maybe that was it, the missing clue.

"Beatriz," I said, "look at the picture that is materializing. This extraordinary home, your whole elegant lifestyle, has come from *your* talent and *your* accomplishments! I see a very different scenario now."

"What do you mean?"

"I imagine the dynamic in your relationship must have changed enormously when you were 'discovered'! Your husband had been the one on the fast track to accolades and then, quite unexpectedly and suddenly, you eclipsed him. Could he have felt overshadowed? Perhaps displaced from his role in

your partnership by your success? That could be a major blow
to his sense of identity, to say nothing of his ego."

Beatriz stared with intense attention, her eyes telling me to
go on, to get to the point.

"And then, a few months ago, COVID changed everything.
Art became secondary, and overnight his work became urgent,
of the highest importance. He goes from feeling left behind to
having the chance to help save all humankind! A chance that
might offer him some of the importance that *you* have enjoyed
for years."

Beatriz's eyes were fixed on me, her head nodding slightly.

"So, if this is right," I continued, "the mystery is suddenly
less mysterious."

"That is . . . very different than I'd thought," she said with
a long sigh.

"It's very different than I'd thought as well," I said. "I'm a
bit . . . more than a bit . . . embarrassed to admit my initial hunch,
that perhaps he was having an affair with another woman."

Her eyes opened wide for a moment. "That would be an interesting twist!"

"Apparently I was off base there," I said, as much a question
as a statement.

"I think so," she said.

"I'm going out on a limb a little here, I admit. But we only
have this one session together, so let's consider what might be
going on now. If my guess is correct, I imagine he is grasping
at this unique opportunity for great success. That motivation
drives him to work at this extraordinary pace. To save you, your
daughter, everyone. And, in so doing, perhaps gain greatness,
fame, wealth. And, maybe most important, your admiration."

Beatriz stared hard as I spoke. After a moment taking this
in, she asked, "So where does that leave me?"

"Learning to be patient, I suspect."

"But what can I do? Do I share these thoughts with him?"

Marilyn's face came to me again, and I thought back to that fraught time. It wasn't the same, but we'd worked it out and learned to evolve our relationship.

"I encourage you to give this new way of looking at things some time. You don't need to do anything right away. Certainly you don't need to jump to suggesting divorce in a crowded restaurant! Support him more, maybe, so he won't feel blamed. And as you get used to this shift in your understanding, you will probably become more comfortable. Then you can share your feelings with him and help him talk about his. If you can do that without taking his responses too personally, without getting too defensive, that will help. It always does."

Several weeks later, I received an email from Beatriz. Our session had completely changed the way she understood her husband's drive. And while it was hard for her not to feel blamed, they were now much better able to speak about their challenges. She felt stronger and, little by little, their relationship was becoming stronger and more tender as well.

What of my experiment with self-disclosure, telling Beatriz the story of my rift with Marilyn those many years ago? The session with Beatriz had been rich and layered, and this story from my life had not been the only source of change. But I suspect it had been a catalyst for her opening up. It certainly hadn't gotten in the way of therapy and likely had accelerated her own disclosure. This was no full-fledged clinical experiment, and there was no useful control group. Nonetheless I decided to keep looking actively for opportunities in which revealing more about myself might help my patients open up.

CHAPTER 12

Albert's Anxiety

A lbert, a physicist in South Africa, emailed requesting a consultation. A few hours before our meeting, I received this email:

The most essential point I wish to discuss is my fear of death. Since I was a child of eight or nine years, the knowledge of the finiteness of my existence has hit me like a lightning bolt. It has been part of my life since then every day every night—more and more since last year when I turned seventy.

It makes sense that people like Albert seek me out, not only because of my long work on existential concerns but also because our culture does such a poor job of dealing with death. We hide it away, replacing it with euphemism ("passing away," "going to a better place," or, as I heard recently from my grandson Adrian, "becoming unalived"), and with stories of eternal life we encounter from folklore and religion alike. Of course the idea of death can certainly be terrifying, but I have no doubt that we exacerbate these fears by collectively burying our heads in the sand. Dying, the one thing that every single one of us will experience, should feature prominently in the way we understand living. I believe that anxiety about death is central to many of the concerns people come to therapy for. Most often this existential fear is buried in the subconscious and manifests in many other ways, often reluctance to engage fully in life—for if one never really lives, one has no real life to lose!—or, conversely, efforts to thumb one's nose at mortality through death-defying feats like skydiving or constantly seeking the excitement of sexual union. I have often encountered these death anxiety–related tendencies in my patients, and have helped many of them manage these fears without being overcome by them.

While this was familiar territory, I was unsure how much I would have to offer Albert in one session. Serious existential work takes time, as fears of death are deeply rooted and intertwined with our ways of living. At the very least, I thought, I could offer some perspectives that had been helpful to other patients, and perhaps share some of my own recent experiences of staring death straight in the eye.

As Albert and I faced each other on Zoom, I saw a thoughtful, energetic, white-haired man. "Professor Yalom," he began, "I'm delighted to meet with you. I'm a professor of physics and please allow me to say something I have not said to anyone for decades: I've long been a student of your work and I am thrilled at the opportunity to meet you face-to-face."

That stopped me for a moment. I'd never met a physicist who was familiar with my work.

"Shall we be informal and use first names?" I asked. "You, 'Albert,' and me, 'Irv'?"

"How about 'Professor' and 'Professor'?" he said. "Just kidding. By all means, first names, I prefer it. It might be a bit awkward for me at first. You've been my teacher for years and I've read many of your books and followed you on Facebook. Or at least I try to. You rarely post."

"True. I did for a while, but I found it consumed too much time. Today, however, we have an entire hour together, so let's plunge right in. You mentioned death anxiety in your email. Can you describe your experience?"

"Hmm. To be honest, this is a first-time occasion. I've never shared this with anyone, not even with my wife. I'm not sure how to start."

"Let me help. Do you remember when you first experienced death anxiety?"

"Oh. I didn't anticipate that question. Let me think."

After closing his eyes and concentrating for a minute, Albert finally said, "One very strong memory surfaces. When I was about eight, I went to my grandfather's funeral, and I remember seeing my father weeping. I tugged on his arm and asked, 'What happens to you after you die?' I guess my father wanted to comfort me (and maybe himself), so he said, 'When you die, you go into a dream state in which you continue to live your life over and over throughout eternity.' I know now that my father was trying to help, but when I was eight it had the opposite effect: it made me feel worse. I was confused by his answer and I asked myself (and my father) over and over, 'How do I know whether my life right now is real or just the dream state?' That thought, that our lives might simply be a dream, has haunted me my whole life. Such irony! What was meant to console me ended up creating so much more anxiety.

"Eventually my father grew annoyed with my questions," Albert continued. "He urged me to simply accept the Church's view of death and the afterlife. I tried for years to believe in the Church's teachings," Albert went on, "but, as I matured and developed a scientist's mind, I concluded that the religious view of afterlife was not supported by any evidence. Long ago, in my early twenties, I left the Church for good, and I've never looked back."

He paused, uttered a few more words, and found he didn't have much more to say. After a bit it was clear that he was having great difficulty recalling any more about the development of his death anxiety. Given the time pressure, I pushed forward. "Perhaps it would be helpful to you if I talked about my own experience with death anxiety."

Albert looked startled. "I'd be most interested. That will probably help my own recall."

"As you may know, my wife died almost exactly a year ago."

"Yes, I read the news of your loss. I'm sorry I did not offer you my condolences. I was unsure of the proper thing to say. In fact, let me be honest. I have a problem speaking to you today. I worry that saying the wrong thing, about death or my fear of it, might cause you pain."

"On the contrary, I prefer your being straightforward, Albert. I find that facing mortality and discussing it openly with others seems to help me. I have been reflecting a great deal on my death anxiety, and it is good to be able to share what I'm learning."

"What have you learned? I'm eager to know."

Hmmm. What *had* I learned? Death has been front and center in my mind ever since Marilyn had been diagnosed with multiple myeloma. During her last few weeks of life she and I had endless talks about death. I'd even reread much of what I'd written about death and our fears of dying in the past. What had helped?

"Well first, I'm learning that writing about death and dying is very different from actually experiencing it," I began. "To be honest, some of the things I've long thought are useful defenses against death anxiety haven't helped me a lot. But others really have. Most important is this: as Marilyn's illness progressed, we agreed over and over that we had few regrets about how we had lived our lives. In fact, even now, I can almost hear her saying, 'The death of an eighty-seven-year-old woman, who lived her life fully, who had four wonderful children and a loving husband always by her side, is not a tragedy.'

"This has really solidified a formula regarding the relationship between how one lives and how one views death. It goes like this: *The fewer regrets about how one has lived, the less death anxiety one experiences.* This is not a new thought. In fact, it's one I've often offered patients. But it has certainly acquired a new relevance for me as my relationship with death has become more . . . intimate. I believe this formula has some power. I wonder, might it have resonance for you?"

Albert closed his eyes in deep concentration for a short time, then shook his head. "I'm not certain that formula works for me, Irv. I've had a good life and few regrets. I've enjoyed my work, I've been creative, I've trained many good students, I've been in love with my wife for nearly fifty years, and I have a wonderful daughter who lives only a couple of kilometers away. Nevertheless, I continue to be haunted by death anxiety, especially the last ten years. Again and again, I've sought help from knowledgeable friends, colleagues, and priests, but always in vain. Honestly, I envy those who are comforted by their religious beliefs, but I just can't believe something I know to be false."

"Your envy of religious believers resonates with me, Albert. Let me tell you about an experience I had recently. I awoke one morning with only a few remnants of a dream about my wife, and I ached with grief, missing her more than ever. Then, from out of nowhere, the thought occurred to me that when I died *I would be buried next to her and thus would be joining Marilyn*. Now, of course, to a rational scientific mind, the idea of *joining Marilyn* is absurd. Marilyn is dead. She no longer exists. And when I die, I will no longer exist. Like you, I have long rejected any religious beliefs of an afterlife. And yet when I thought about *joining Marilyn*, anxiety flowed out of me and comfort flowed in, seeping through my body. Strange, isn't it—that I can somehow *know* one thing in my rational mind and simultaneously have a powerful emotional response to the opposite idea?"

"Very strange," Albert agreed.

"Well, we are human and can hold contradictions. This one illuminates for me the remarkable gift that religion offers," I continued. "It makes me appreciate how every major religion has, in one way or another, offered humankind the solace of continued existence. How comforting that would be."

Albert nodded. "It almost makes me wish I could believe."

"Almost."

"May I ask a personal question? I gather from your writing that you are an atheist, but also that you grew up in a traditional Jewish household. How did you lose, or escape, religion?"

"It never made sense to me," I said. "You're right that my childhood world was *very* Jewish. My parents had fled the Old World in the 1920s and ended up in Washington, DC, with a group of others from the same shtetl, Seltz, a speck on the map in the old Russian Empire. But many hadn't made it— siblings, cousins, friends—and had died in the Nazi camps. This shadow hung over our whole community. In any case, my parents spoke Yiddish, everything I ate was kosher, and I hardly knew anyone who wasn't Jewish. Culturally it seemed normal. But I couldn't fathom the religion. Was my eating a cheeseburger truly something that would offend a God who was busy taking care of the entire universe? Like you, I have a strong memory of an important encounter with my father. We were having lunch together one day and I remember asking him if he believed in God. 'After the Shoah, how can anyone believe in God?' he responded. That finally sealed it for me."

Was all this information helpful for Albert? I didn't know, and talking about the Holocaust certainly wasn't likely to ease anyone's anxiety. But he had asked for my history, and I did not see any harm in sharing it.

"Thank you, Irv," he said after taking all of this in. "It's helpful to hear that you have struggled with this, too."

"Albert, let me return to the question I asked a few minutes ago. Please focus as deeply as you can on the formula that the fewer regrets about how one lived, the less death anxiety one experiences. Does that have any meaning to you?"

Albert pondered for a moment. He responded, "I've been considering it, but I don't think so. I am haunted by death anxiety and yet I feel no regrets. Professionally I've had a career that far exceeded anything I dreamed of doing. I researched and wrote, influenced my field heavily. I received many important prizes. I've had a good life."

"So, my linkage of regrets and death anxiety doesn't resonate for you? That's important for me to know."

"No, no, wait. Let's not rush to that conclusion. It's a new concept and I'm searching for a way to explore."

Albert wore a lovely expression of intense curiosity as he turned the idea over in his mind. I watched, enthralled, for a couple of moments, until it seemed he was stuck.

"Try this," I said. "Just concentrate on the phrase *regrets in my life*, and then think aloud for a couple of minutes. Simply say whatever comes into your mind. Omit nothing, censor nothing, force nothing."

"Hmmm. I'll give it a try. Never done this before . . . get loose . . . don't think, just speak . . . demanding father . . . he darkened our lives . . . much regret at not having had a loving father . . . he poisoned the whole family . . . my two brothers were deeply scarred by him—I was the youngest and least damaged—he died when I was twelve . . . so, yes, regrets about my family whenever I see a loving, happy family." He paused. "Is this what you mean, Irv?"

"Exactly. Keep going."

"But once I grew into an adult and left the family home, I've had no real regrets. Quite the opposite. Hmmm . . . married forty-eight years—good marriage—wonderful daughter, always loved my wife—maybe a few regrets about not playing the field longer . . . about not having sexual adventures before marriage. . . . And regrets about my son . . . unable to find himself professionally and unable to find a good mate." Albert stopped and looked at me. "Is this okay? I sort of switched."

"You're doing great. I know this is not easy, but try to continue for just a couple more minutes."

Albert nodded and took a deep breath. "Regrets . . . well, yes, yes, I have to acknowledge many regrets about my wife's health . . . she was so often sick, couldn't travel . . . we never could take vacation trips . . . migraine and asthma . . . and every time we tried to travel she got sick . . . I never stopped loving her but, yes, regrets . . . all the trips we never took . . . all the things we could have done and were unable to . . . hard to even have friends over for dinner . . . some anger there for sure. . . . Dr. Yalom, facing myself in this manner is not easy. I'm exhausted."

"How could you not be? You've just done some amazing

work, and I'm honored you've trusted me so much. Let's review what's happened in the last few minutes. At first, when
you posited that you had no significant regrets, I couldn't help
feeling that there was a darkened room in the house of your
mind that you avoid entering. And then, when you did open it
and turned on the light, regrets poured out: about your father's
destructive influence on you and your brothers. And then you
spoke of your son, and your wife and her illness, and all the
experiences you and she never had."

"Yes. I wasn't really aware that all that was there. Surprising.
And I feel a bit guilty admitting those things."

"This is important, Albert. Let me emphasize that having
regrets, even many regrets, even anger, about the life you and
your wife have lived is *not* incompatible with loving her, loving
her very deeply. The same with your son. Both things can be
true."

"I'm shivering as you say that. I wish we could continue to
meet and explore the last idea."

"Albert, I'd love to. I just don't have the memory or the
stamina. But remember, you are human and can hold contradictions. Just as you felt that shiver, I urge you to investigate
these thoughts, ideally with one of the therapists I'll refer you
to. This won't magically cure all of your anxiety about death,
but it's certainly where I would start exploring. And it may
help you see where you want to put your energies in your life
now."

With Albert looking surprised and exhausted, we wished
each other well and said goodbye. As I clicked "end meeting"
and my screen darkened, I reviewed our session in my mind.
I was pleased. I had been helpful—of that I had no doubt.
I had shared my inner thoughts with him, my thoughts on
religion and my memory of my father, as well as my relief at

"joining Marilyn." I believe the observations about religion had cemented a bond between us as fellow skeptics, building a certain intellectual alliance. And opening up about "joining Marilyn" and my own ambivalence toward the comforting con game of religious belief revealed my own vulnerability, and likely helped build an emotional bridge between us. This seemed like another successful use of explicit, intentional self-disclosure. Each time I had offered some bit of my inner world in a consultation, it had helped my patient open up and quickly brought the two of us closer.

But I have my limits, and there are some things I am not sharing. What I did not tell Albert was that, earlier in the day, my daughter set off for a thirty-minute walk to the cemetery to visit my wife's burial site. As always, she invited me to join her and, as always, I declined. Marilyn died a year before, but I still hadn't visited her grave, not once. Whenever I thought of her or saw a picture of her, I continued to feel a stab in the heart. Was that why I declined? Or was it because I chose not to see the empty plot next to her, the plot where I will soon be buried? I really don't know.

I do think a lot about dying these days, but I rarely find myself overwhelmed by fear or anxiety. It is more a presence that shows up, insists on sticking around and conversing, and then fades away. My willingness to sit with this presence despite the discomfort, to accept the inevitability of death, and to look at it squarely over the years is, I'm certain, an important reason why I no longer find it terrifying.

CHAPTER 13

Sparring with Serenity, Dueling with Trauma

S oon after Albert, another patient reached out to me with uncomfortable thoughts about death. Antje's tranquil face appeared on my screen, seeming only a few feet away though I was in California and she was in her Berlin apartment nearly six thousand miles away. The connection was excellent. No bad audio, glitchy video, or faulty hearing aids to worry about. Here a chill permeated the air as November set in. I suspect it was already bitingly cold in Germany, yet Antje's room seemed bathed in warm, golden light.

"Good to see you, Dr. Yalom," she began. "I know your face well from your author photos." She pointed her computer toward her bookcase so that I could see several of my books in German translation.

"I like your taste in literature, Antje. Tell me, was there something in particular in my writing that prompted you to contact me now?"

"Your existential perspective, I suspect. I've been tormented recently by a deluge of obsessive thoughts about death," she responded, leaning back into her seat.

As I mentioned before, I have worked for decades with many patients dealing with existential anxieties. I am even guilty of steering some patients who enter therapy with seemingly un-related concerns into the existential realm. In light of Marilyn's passing, and my own looming mortality, these patients' con-cerns seemed even more pressing. I felt both armed with new perspectives that might be helpful and cautious, perhaps a bit reluctant, to look as closely as I might have when I was younger and more vital.

"Is this a new experience for you," I asked Antje, "these thoughts of death?"

"Hmmm . . . yes. I imagine COVID is responsible. This quarantine really rubs it in one's face, mortality, doesn't it?"

"Good insight," I said. "So these invasive thoughts began during quarantine?"

"Well . . . now that you have me thinking about it, I've had them occasionally since my mother committed suicide seven years ago. But they are much stronger lately."

"Can you describe them for me?"

"Here's an example. I'm with my boyfriend, Klaus. We spend most of our nights together and I like him very much. He's my age, thirty-one, and we're having a good time together, say having drinks and maybe watching a film. And then some voice, coming from some dark part of me, softly but firmly reminds me that we are all going to die. I'm going to die, and Klaus is going to die, and everyone we know, and there's no point at all to life."

She made a soft gesture with her hand, opening her fingers as if they were the petals of a dandelion blowing off into the wind, *poof*, then lifted a tall glass of juice or perhaps iced tea to her lips and took a slow sip.

"I try not to talk about it with him," she continued. "It just poisons our time. At least for me. But those dark words inside my head are growing louder and louder."

As I listened to Antje, I was struck by the contrast between her words and her tone. Her words were dark, bleak, and yet everything else about her—her posture, her face—was languid and peaceful. I felt like an interloper splashing boorishly in a pool of tranquility.

"And when you hear that other voice, that dark voice you can't turn off, how do you handle it?"

"Sometimes I do end up telling Klaus. It doesn't bother him. He's very cool. Mostly I just try to ignore it. Think about other things. But no matter how hard I try, I can't entirely force it from my mind. I do *not* want it there. Can you help with that?"

"Well, let's get to work. What impact does this have on your relationship with Klaus?"

"As I say, Klaus just flows with it. He's very cool about everything."

I waited for more, but she seemed content, a calm smile playing on her lips.

"Tell me more about your relationship with him. How long has it been?"

"We've been together for six years."

"Your thoughts about the future?"

"Why bring up the future? We're too young, too busy enjoying life. We inhabit the *here and now*, as you often put it in your writing."

"Enjoying life. That's a nice place to be, Antje."

I was perplexed. She was letting me know she needed help,

yet she exuded such extraordinary placidity. This strong contrast between words and demeanor usually indicates that something is askew, that the problem the patient has identified is not the whole story. It was my task to dig into her discomfort and see what else might be there. I strode onward.

"But then, here you are, calling me. Why?"

"These damned death thoughts are getting worse. I've done three twelve-week courses of cognitive behavioral therapy, but it hasn't really helped. Nothing has changed. I have several friends who are therapists, and they urged me to contact you. So here I am. Can you help get rid of these thoughts?"

She said this so matter-of-factly, as if it were a supremely simple request, like yanking out a bad tooth. Then she took another slow sip from her drink. She had a deep concern that must be a bit frightening to share with me, the doctor of last resort. Yet I couldn't help feeling like she was relaxing at a beachfront bar. I dove further in.

"Antje, let's go back to the very beginning of these obsessions. Tell me how and when they started."

"With my mother's suicide, as I said. About seven years ago." She smiled again and brushed some hair from her face.

"Tell me more about your parents."

"They divorced when I was a young child. I have no memory of the three of us living together. My father bought a house two blocks away from my mother's, and I spent every other evening with him. Even now I spend a couple of evenings with my father every week—Klaus is entirely cool with that. But back to my mother. She had serious problems. She was bipolar—sometimes she loved me, sometimes she was too depressed to even notice I was there. She was hospitalized more times than I can count."

"And when she *was* at home, what was she like?"

"Distant. Troubled. She wasn't all there, you know? I don't have memories of her caring for me. She couldn't really take care of herself. Yes, that's the truth."

Though her smile was as mellow as ever, I was certain this was a delicate topic and I tried to be gentle. "Can you say just a bit more about that? In which ways couldn't she take care of herself?"

"Making food, cleaning the house, all the basics. The place was a mess, and I had to fend for myself. Also, she was a klep-tomaniac. A clumsy one, I guess, because she got arrested for stealing all the time and was in jail for weeks or months at a go. She was into drugs, too, using and selling. Seven years ago she died from a heroin overdose. Was it an accident? My father and I consider it suicide, but who knows?"

Imagine, having a mother who was absent at best, unable to offer the basic protections of parenthood. It must have been frightening. I wanted to gather more information about her harrowing childhood and allow it to be present with us, but I knew that it was important to tread softly here. Moving too fast risked reopening deep wounds, and doing so without the time to treat those wounds would be irresponsible. I went on, cautiously.

"So for a number of years there were just the two of you in the house and it seems unclear who was the child and who the mother?"

"Well, as I mentioned, my father's house was just a couple of blocks away and I often stayed with him. It was supposed to be every other night but actually I spent way more than fifty percent of the time there. Not just when my mother was in jail or the hospital, but because he was a wonderful father. That's something else I should say, which is that my dark death thoughts are not just about me or Klaus. Often they are about my father dying. I really love him, and this worries me all the time."

I was glad to hear of her strong bond with her father and had the impulse to let her continue talking about him. But there was no time to meander, and I chose to steer toward the discomfort of her mother, feeling there likely was more paydirt in that difficult relationship.

"Antje, can you tell me what it felt like to be in your mother's house?"

"I'm not sure how this is important. I mean, that was a long, very long, time ago. And things are so much better. What I need is your help with these invasive thoughts I'm having now! Can you help me with these existential issues? Other therapists have failed and now I turn to you."

There was that challenge again: *please fix me!* But she didn't want to talk about the future and wouldn't dig further into the past. Somehow neither of these connected to the "here and now" of her excellent relationship with Klaus, movie nights with languorous beverages, and the haunting invasive thoughts. I thought about her significant childhood trauma, and the ever-cool Klaus seemed to make sense. Perhaps she needed someone whom she could rely on but who was also just detached enough that she would not have to be *too* close, *too* intimate with. Real intimacy can be a double-edged sword for those of us carrying such trauma. We crave closeness but are also wary of it, as we've been hurt, abandoned, or neglected before.

How to get beyond her serene surface and really connect? I reached once again for self-disclosure, hoping to quickly bypass some of her defenses, and was curious how this approach would work.

"Antje, let me tell you a story about my wife, Marilyn, and

me. Nature conducted an interesting experiment for us. At
first it may not seem related to your situation, but hear me
out and you'll see why I'm telling this to you. Here's a quick
summary: Her parents and my parents emigrated from Poland
and Russia, respectively, to Washington, DC, shortly after
World War I. Our parents did not know one another, even
though her father opened a grocery store on Second and Seaton Street and my father opened a store just a block away at
First and Seaton. In fact, the first time they met each other
was at our wedding, but that's another story.

"My father had decided that our family should live directly
over the store, so for the first fourteen years of my life I spent
my time in a run-down apartment in a dangerous neighborhood, while my parents worked downstairs twelve hours a day.
Washington was heavily segregated then, and we were the
only Jewish family in a poor Black neighborhood. I wasn't allowed to be friends with any of those kids. The cultural divide
was too wide for my parents, and probably for me, too. And the
white kids screamed anti-Semitic slurs at me whenever they
saw me. So I was mostly alone, and often scared.

"Everything changed in ninth grade, when my mother
bought us a house in a nicer part of town, just a few blocks
from Marilyn's home. Her father had made a very different
choice than mine. He thought the neighborhood by the stores
was too dangerous for his three girls to grow up in, so he
had purchased a modest house for his family in a safer part
of Washington and commuted twenty minutes to work each
day. Marilyn never set foot in her father's store and spent her
childhood without fear. She had a great many friends and
took elocution and piano and dancing and French lessons.

"Now, Antje, here's the reason I'm telling you this: these
first fourteen years left indelible marks upon us. Marilyn was

sheltered, cherished, and surrounded by a large cohort of admiring friends and teachers. She never experienced anxiety. *She didn't know what anxiety was,* and she grew up calm, graceful, and self-assured. I, on the other hand, have been plagued by anxiety throughout my life, a constant, dreadful companion that I've never been able to fully shake. Several rounds of therapy have been quite helpful, but I'm still often haunted by unbidden thoughts, by images that creep into my dreams or feelings of sudden discomfort."

Noting Antje's puzzled look, I commented, "This is a long story, and you must be wondering why I'm telling it now. I feel it has great relevance to you. All the available research in our field strongly indicates that an early, unsafe environment, like the one you experienced with your mother, leaves an imprint, a dark persistent imprint. Do you see where I'm heading?"

"I think so. But, as I've told you, that part of my life is long past. Long-forgotten past history. Life is good now."

"Antje, please trust me when I say that early history is *not* forgotten. Remember those horrific thoughts that keep coasting into your mind? Yes, you've made a good life for yourself, with a caring partner. But realize that who you are is not simply this person existing in the present moment. We are all made up of our experiences and our memories and our dreams, and our brains and nervous systems have a way of holding on to all of this experience. So while we might be able to push them out of our consciousness, these past traumas find ways to seep in. That dark voice was born in your early years. Those thoughts are why you're now asking for my help."

She mulled this over for a moment.

"I really don't want to think about all of that. Things are fine now."

Again she pushed back. She clearly did not want to accept

that dealing with the voices that were plaguing her might require digging through her traumatic past. I understood that
resistance, but I only had a short time to be helpful. I shifted
into the here and now.

"Let me ask you a different question, Antje. How are you
and I doing in this session today?"

"Well, I've been happy to be able to unload these dark
thoughts to you. But I really can't understand why you keep
tying these fleeting feelings back to my childhood. Honestly, I
feel like you're not responding to what I'm asking, which is to
help me get rid of them!"

"Maybe telling you my experience of our session will be
helpful."

"Okay."

"You wonder why I keep tying these aspects of your past together with what is happening for you in the present. Let me
be very direct, as we only have this one hour together. You've
asked me for help, and I know from long experience that
the types of childhood trauma you're describing—a chaotic
and hazardous early life, an upbringing where you never received the consistent love and protection that young children
require—these things often manifest later in life in anxiety
around death. I've encountered versions of this many times.
And yet every time I try to make that connection, you raise
some defenses and push it away. Ironically, perhaps, your
strong resistance to talking about your childhood strengthens
my belief that we are on to a very difficult area that needs to
be explored."

"But it really doesn't feel related to how things are now."

"Maybe you're right, and maybe I'm way off base here, Antje.
But let me ask, why are you dismissing the idea so quickly
rather than having some curiosity around this possibility?"

"That period just feels so . . . dark. That's not what my life feels like now."

"Yes, from the very onset of our talk today I've been struck by your serenity, Antje. I've admired it, even envied it. And I have no doubt that this calm demeanor has made you more comfortable in the world and more liked and accepted by your friends. But I also suspect this is your way of protecting yourself from dreadful memories."

On the screen, from a continent away, Antje's eyes were tightly fixated on me. "Okay," she said slowly, with a hint of a question.

"I think you've tried very hard to keep them out of your awareness."

"My previous therapist never asked much about my childhood."

"This is uncomfortable. But please believe me when I say that short, behaviorally focused efforts to change your thinking, like the courses of CBT you mentioned, are not going to give you the help you need."

"So, what are you suggesting?"

"I'm suggesting an entirely different approach to therapy for you. These early life memories are painful and, as ample research has shown, extremely hard to erase or ignore. Fortunately a great deal of progress in understanding trauma like ours, and developing methods of treating it, has been made in recent years. I'm suggesting longer-term work with a therapist focusing on early childhood trauma. Together you can confront, explore, and ultimately work through these memories."

She began to speak, then paused, wrestling with the idea of looking directly where she did not want to look. After a moment she spoke up again.

"So reframing the thoughts when they come up is not a good approach?"

"It won't stop them from coming. They are rooted much deeper. Also, and here's a difficult aspect, these are not simple cognitive distortions. Your *panic* about death needs to be addressed, but the thoughts have truth in them. We *are* all going to die, you and Klaus, eventually. And much sooner, me. How we can live most richly during the time we have seems to me the most important question. For you, exploring your early trauma, and these existential thoughts, with a good therapist over time, should help."

Antje's lovely smile had vanished. "Tell me more about the work you think I need to do in long-term therapy."

Her curiosity struck me as a hopeful sign. I wanted to make therapy feel both critical and inviting. And I wanted to give her enough understanding of trauma treatment to make good decisions, without overloading her with information.

"Antje, all this pain from your past will not stay buried and can't simply be ignored. In therapy you'll look at these memories and experiences carefully, think about how they show up elsewhere in your thinking and how they've impacted you. Ideally you'll go slowly, at whatever pace you can tolerate. Also, deep trauma like yours has a significant component that isn't cognitive or intellectual. It resides deeper in the nervous system, and there are somatic modalities, and EMDR, which works with eye movements and patterns of tapping, which your therapist may want to use in concert with talk therapy to help retrain parts of your nervous system. I imagine at least a year of therapy, which may seem like a long time to explore uncomfortable things. But, if you do persevere, I am convinced that it will be enormously helpful to you."

Antje nodded. Her serene smile was gone. Her once placid

eyes now brimmed with such fear and worry that I was reluctant to end our hour. "I know this has not been easy for you, Antje. I'm digging up painful memories that you've wanted to forget. But, trust me, working with one of the therapists I'll recommend will make a major difference in your life."

She whispered a barely audible "Thank you" as she signed off, looking nothing like the confident, peaceful woman she'd been an hour ago.

Hours later, Antje's frightened face remained in my mind. I had once again been quite direct. I'd pointed out her strong resistance much sooner than I would have in my more accustomed, longer-term therapy, perhaps well before she felt she could trust me fully. Of course it was possible that my interpretation was wrong, that her invasive thoughts about death were not rooted in her childhood trauma but resulted from some other, more recent life experience. I had, once again, been quite directive, insisting on the connections between her childhood trauma and her present fears, rather than helping her see the connections for herself. But there had been no time!

I tried to reassure myself that I had done the right thing. I strongly believed that it was imperative for her to do deep work on herself, to uncover and face the demons of her early trauma. Still, this consultation was not easy to dismiss. I am always uncomfortable when a patient ends a session more upset than they were at the onset.

Several weeks later, I emailed Antje, inquiring about how she was doing. She responded quite happily that her intrusive existential fears had ceased after we spoke. She realized there was still denial at play but that she'd been significantly less troubled since then. I was relieved that I hadn't sent her further into crisis. But she also noted that she did not feel she needed further therapy at this time. I feared she had slipped back behind her curtain of serenity. And yet she had so much work to do, if she could only overcome her imperturbable resistance! I quickly wrote back:

> Hi, Antje,
> I'm pleased to know that you're doing well. Even so, I want to repeat my advice to enter ongoing therapy. Let's consider it prophylaxis—something to ensure that these dark voices of your anxiety will not haunt you in the future. Trust me on this. As I mentioned, I, too, had a difficult early life, and my own therapy has been invaluable.
> Please check in again in the future.
>
> My best wishes, Antje
>
> —Irv Yalom

And that was as far as I could take it. I very much hope she has found her way to exploring those dark corners, but it's likely I will never know.

What of my disclosing my stories about my childhood and Marilyn's, nature's experiment with anxiety? Had this served Antje well? I was not sure. It had certainly brought the topic of Antje's childhood trauma to the forefront and made it easier to talk about. And perhaps in telling the story I'd given myself trauma bona fides, as it were. But she hadn't been fully ready to confront how her past was impacting her present, regardless of how urgently I had pushed.

Had I pushed too hard? I wasn't sure. She had experienced some relief after our session and, even if it were temporary, that was a good thing. On the other hand, our session certainly made Antje uncomfortable, and the idea of undergoing longer-term uncomfortable self-exploration may have deterred her from seeking helpful therapy. Moving forward I would be cautious when I felt myself becoming too directive. It often seemed necessary in the short time frame, but I'd need to remind myself to proceed with caution.

CHAPTER 14

Tough Love

Dr. Yalom—

I'm a forty-five-year-old psychiatrist in rural Texas. Many of my patients travel long distances to see me and I feel that I should be learning more to help them. I love my work, but I've been stagnating the last few years. I go to conferences and lectures with the hopes of learning something new, but the phony speakers only offer the same stale crap. My peers call me for help when they're stuck, and I always help them. Now I'm the one feeling stuck, but no one ever has anything I haven't figured out already.

I was first introduced to you by a memorable professor who required Love's Executioner *in his course. I followed that book with your others, and they were all helpful— every damned one of them! But now I feel stuck in the mud and I don't like it. I want to keep growing. Can I have a consultation with you?*

Gene

I am always interested when a therapist wants to give more to his patients, and I responded proposing an appointment three weeks later. When Gene's face appeared on my screen, I was startled. I guess I'd been thinking of Gene Autry, the cowboy movie star and country singer who had been so popular when I was a kid. That, coupled with the rough language of the email, had me expecting a tough old codger with a few days of stubble and a missing front tooth or two. Instead, facing me was a broad-shouldered woman who wore a plaid shirt and had pale blue eyes and straight white teeth.

"Good to meet you, Gene. I know you are feeling stuck. Tell me more."

"Well, I'm the therapist other therapists around here turn to when they don't know what else to do. Maybe you've had that, too? Folks know goddamn well there ain't nothing I can't handle—everything from alcoholics and wife-beating a-holes to bipolar folks, schizophrenics, and the beaten wives of the aforementioned a-holes."

"Sounds like you know what you're doing."

"I sure as hell do!" she said, with a toothy smile. "I find solutions, and I don't take crap from anyone!"

"And the stuckness?"

"Not exactly sure how to put it. Something about wanting to do more. Or maybe go deeper. Does that make sense? I'm damn good at getting people to stop doing stupid things. Stop hurting themselves or others, stop messing up their families— that kind of thing. But with a lot of cases it's just problem solving."

"Instead of what?"

"Something more lasting, I guess. Like a guy comes to me with a problem. Okay, I can help him find his way through that usually. But often that feels like that kid with his finger in the dike. I know the same problem is going to pop up again, maybe in a different place in his life, or a different shape, in a couple of years. Ya' know what I mean?"

"I think I do, Gene. You want to give them something more impactful, something that gets at the root causes of their behavior maybe."

"Yes. Exactly. It's frustrating."

"Do you talk to anyone about this? Colleagues?"

"Like I said in my email, it doesn't seem like anyone here ever has much to offer. Nothing I haven't already figured out through trial and error. Or reading."

"That's tough. I've always needed colleagues to talk to. But maybe that was easier for me to find, being at a major university."

"Not much of that out here."

Having people to discuss ideas with has always been important to me, from my colleagues in the department at Stanford, to therapist support groups, to the writers' group I've been part of for decades. I thought how hard it would be not to have these peers to share my challenges with. Then I realized that I'd heard versions of this from some of my Silicon Valley patients. Perhaps sharing this would be helpful.

"Gene," I said, "I've worked with a number of really successful people over the years. They often relate some version of how lonely it is to be at the top, to be the one making decisions. There's no one to share the weight with. I wonder if a bit of this is at play for you."

"Suppose I could talk over my cases with the cattle," she said with a short laugh. She gazed off to the side, maybe looking out a window. "You think that would breach confidentiality?"

I was going to dig further into her practice, but that gaze into the distance gave me the feeling this conversation might not be just about her work.

"Can you tell me a bit about your home life?"

Gene began to fill me in. She lived in a small town, alone. She had been married but had divorced her "horse-assed alcoholic good-for-nothing good-riddance husband" after only three years and had long ago, "thank the good Lord," lost touch with him. She had a horse, whom she rode whenever she could, and a lazy one-eyed dog who followed her everywhere, slowly.

When I asked about children, Gene's voice suddenly softened. "My girl, Justine, my only child, died of leukemia almost a year ago. I guess I'm still mired in deep grief." Gene grabbed a large handkerchief from her rear pocket and blew her nose loudly. Then, in a gentle voice, she said, "Dr. Yalom, I know that you, too, are in mourning for your wife and I need to ask straight out: Are you up to the task of meeting with a tough patient?"

By now I was getting used to Marilyn's death coming up in sessions.

"Honestly it hasn't been easy, but I'm getting help, and I'm healing. You ask if I'm up to the task. From the standpoint of empathy and understanding your experience, I just might be the ideal consultant for you."

"I get that. You've been down this road and you just might know the way back home."

"Yep. On a rough journey it's best to travel with someone by your side. Tell me, Gene, you got someone close? Someone you can lean on? Unload to?" I noticed I was slipping into a bad imitation of her speech. I could imagine myself chewing tobacco by the end of our hour if I weren't careful.

Gene had a hard time with my question. She looked flustered, searched for words, and then, quietly, said, "I had a good friend. Ellen. Tough as nails. We used to go skydiving and did lots of big game hunting together. But, shit, she moved away years ago—to Utah to be a grandmother to her son's kids. Can you believe that? I've lost touch with her. I won't lie. The truth is, it hurts to even talk about her. I've never replaced her. Someone close, you ask?" She shook her head a bit sadly. "No one else."

"And, of course," I added, "with COVID, connecting is harder than ever. The isolation can wear you down."

She nodded, then stayed quiet in thought. After a couple of minutes she surprised me by switching roles and taking the proverbial reins of the conversation. "Let me ask more about how you're faring, Irv. I know your wife and my girl died about the same time."

I welcomed her invitation to speak more intimately but also knew this might be a deflection away from her own pain. I saw two options: I could continue questioning her about intimacy or I could model an intimate experience for her. I picked the latter without hesitation.

"I'm finding grief is a tough trip. Our relationship was pretty unusual. I met Marilyn when I was fourteen years old. Bottom line, we were inseparable for seventy-four years. I've never known a friend, or a patient, or, for that matter, anyone, who had that long a bond. When she died, I knew enough about grief to realize my prognosis was not good. And, indeed, I have not fared that well. I'm still working on it, seeing a good thera- pist, and still hurting. I still can't look at photos of her without feeling a stab in my heart, and I still haven't managed to visit her grave. But I am recovering, slowly."

"How do you do it?" she said. "Grieve?"

"No easy answer. But let me share something, Gene. Recently, I've been rereading some of my own books. Some of them aren't too bad, by the way! I guess it's a way of looking back on my own life. Anyways, a couple of weeks ago I opened a book of stories, *Momma and the Meaning of Life*, and saw a story called 'Eight Advanced Lessons in the Therapy of Grief.' I'm a bit embarrassed to admit this, but my memory is failing and I had completely forgotten writing it. Any chance you remember that one?"

"I loved that book. But I can't recall the story. Sorry."

"It's about a patient of mine, a professor who had recently lost her husband and her brother and who was, understandably, angry at the universe. She was also angry at me for having had such a comfortable, pain-free life. She felt my life was so easy that I couldn't really appreciate what she was going through, and we had serious arguments about this. I remember losing my temper one day and saying, 'So I have to be depressed to treat depression? Or schizophrenic to treat a schizophrenic? Is that what you're saying?' I thought her position was so ridiculous at the time. But now that I'm deep in grief and going through many stages including denial, numbness, obsessional thinking, and so on, I've come to the conclusion that she was right. Now, only now, suffering this pain, do I really know what she was going through. I am a better therapist as a result of it. I don't like the trade-off, but there's a lot to be said for life experience."

I found myself wanting a break, as it was hard to think about Marilyn just then. But Gene pressed on.

"And now? Do you live alone now?"

"Three of my four children live within an hour's drive and each week one of them visits and spends a night or two with me. I have my helper, Joe, who lives in my wife's old studio and helps keep me going. COVID greatly increases my isolation, of course. I'm pushing ninety and doubt I would survive if I caught the virus. Still, most days one of my kids or a friend comes over and we put on masks, take a walk with my trusty walker, and talk together."

"Can I ask you another question?"

"Of course, Gene."

I noticed that she took a deep breath and then, in a softer voice, asked, "How did you make your friends?"

As I've aged I've grown far more emotionally labile, and Gene's gentle question, her opening up this way, brought tears to my eyes. I felt honored by her trusting me and, ignoring my own moistening eyes, responded fully to her question. "I had a small group of friends that I made early in life. Four of them were from med school. There were only five Jews allowed in my class, and in anatomy we were all assigned to one cadaver. We became very close over that somewhat macabre bonding experience and remained lifelong friends. Other than that odd grouping, Marilyn made most of our friends. She was far more social than I, loved dinners and parties and meeting new people. I've always been more awkward. I did become close with some of my students over the years, and they still come to visit and take slow walks with me. Why those ones in particular and not others? I'd say that my friends are all folks who are open, who reveal themselves to me, who are not trying to impress me. I guess those are the factors that encouraged me to be open to them."

We fell silent for a couple of minutes. I thought about how all those friends from my early life were gone now, how I was the last still breathing.

Then I circled back and said, "Gene, as you probably know from my writing, I'm an advocate of examining the here and now and I'd like to share what I've been feeling. A couple of minutes ago you asked me about how I made friends. What I didn't say to you was that I was so touched by your question that tears came to my eyes." I was going to continue but decided to stop at this point in order to bring her even closer.

Gene, puzzled and uncomfortable, shook her head slightly in consternation and looked for a moment as though she were going to speak, then remained silent.

"Gene, can you put the feelings you're having right now into words? Please give it a try."

"Uh, well . . . confused."

"Confused starting when? Can you try to pinpoint it?"

"I'm not good at this but I guess it was when you said something about tears."

"I said that I was moved to tears when you asked me about how I made friends. What did that touch off in you?"

Gene looked decidedly uncomfortable, shrugged her shoulders, and drew her lips together.

"Try once more to put those feelings into words, Gene."

"I don't know . . . tears . . . yuck . . . maybe it was too close . . . I don't want to . . . I don't know how to talk about it."

"So, here's what I've been thinking, Gene. I felt your question about how I made friends was so very important. I was moved by it because it signaled your wish for intimacy. It signaled your saying that you wanted help and you wanted to get closer to me, and to others. I think one of the major issues you need to explore is the bind you're in, between wanting to be a tough, hard-assed cowboy on the one hand and, on the other hand, wanting to express your more tender, sensitive side."

After a long silence I nudged her. "I can't quite hear you, Gene."

She looked distressed and almost whispered, "We're approaching some tough territory. This is a small community and I'm well known for my efficiency. I'm not comfortable revealing soft or vulnerable sides of myself, certainly not to anyone around here."

"Gene, what I'm really asking is that you reveal it to yourself . . . and also to me. Tell me, what's the risk in exploring that part of yourself?"

"Don't know. It's just unknown territory."

"We were in this territory earlier when you talked about your friend Ellen, and again, a few minutes ago, when you asked me about how I made friends and I told you that your question and your wish for closeness touched me so much. That was the moment when I felt really close to you. What about you? What about *your* experience?"

"Yep. Unknown territory for me, and honestly damn scary. I get you. I understand what you're saying, but I can't stay there long. Intimacy, tenderness, softness . . . these are all strangers for me. I never knew them, never felt comfortable with them."

"Let me share something else with you, Gene. At the very beginning of our meeting I was surprised when a woman appeared on my screen. My sister was named Jean, but with the more feminine spelling. The way you write it brought to mind Gene Autry or Gene Kelly, so I was expecting a man to appear on my screen. You've had this man's name all your life. Is this at all relevant to our discussion?"

"Nah, I don't think so. What I was told was that my dad was infatuated with the actress Gene Tierney. But she's the only woman I know of who used that spelling. Having a guy's name never bothered me. I kinda liked it. Still do. I did think about changing it to Loretta when I hit puberty. But I had no one to talk to about it. I never had sisters or close girlfriends. Yeah, now that I think about it, there were a few times I thought about changing my name to a real girl's name but, trust me, in my community being thought of as tough had its advantages."

"Any advantages to letting that other side out?"

"Maybe. Probably worth exploring."

She was tough, but she also seemed willing to explore alternatives. I pushed a bit further, to see if this was just talk, or if she were truly willing to go further.

"Gene, from what you've just shared with me, I get the feeling that you're ready to make some significant changes. How do you feel about entering therapy now?"

"I'm uncomfortable talking about therapy. Even thinking about it, honestly. Which I realize is ridiculous for a therapist. But I'm in a small community where everyone knows everyone, and the gossip runs wild."

"I can understand that problem. Fortunately COVID has this one silver lining: almost all therapists are working virtually now, which means you can see someone who has no connection to your community. Could be individual therapy, could be a group."

Her eyes perked up suddenly. "I hadn't thought of a group. Tell me a bit more how that might work for me."

"What I'm thinking is that you originally contacted me about feeling stuck professionally. But as we got talking, it seems like you're stuck personally, too. You've had this rawhide exterior, which serves you so well as Gene the therapist of last resort who can handle everything. At the same time, maybe it's not serving you so well for Gene the person who, I believe, needs more connection. A good group would be a place to work on learning to connect, and maybe on trying to let that more sensitive side out and seeing how other people respond. I'm glad to email you some therapists, group and individual, to check out."

"I'm game," she responded, "and I will follow through. Thank you, Irv. This session has been a great gift."

Our time was up, and I was about to sign off, but a thought kept pressing at me.

"One last thing, Gene. There were a couple of times during our session when you sort of took the reins, if you know what I mean. You started asking questions about me—How am *I* faring with grief? How did *I* make friends?—rather than letting me, the therapist, ask questions of you. It was pretty unusual. Any thoughts on this?"

She mulled this over for moment, then shrugged with a smile. "I guess I'm just more comfortable leading. Must be the Gene Kelly in me."

Gene told me I'd given her a gift, and I felt strongly that she would make good use of opportunities to explore changes in her life. But I had the feeling that she had given me a gift, too. She said she'd reversed roles because that position was more comfortable for her. I suspect she felt more in control and less vulnerable. But there was something else there, something useful. What if I were to challenge patients explicitly to ask me personal questions? What might that yield?

Of course patients have asked me hundreds of such questions over the years, and there is a great deal to be learned from what a patient chooses to ask. What are they interested in, and what does that reveal about their concerns? Gene had asked how I had made friends, and it was clear that she was struggling with loneliness and a lack of connection. That was valuable information. Beyond this, however, insisting they ask personal questions would require them to get close, to reach out in an intimate way. It would give me the opportunity to model openness and sharing.

Was there danger in having patients ask the questions? Most schools that train psychotherapists would balk at the idea of making the space for such personal inquiry. But what are we afraid our patients are going to ask? Will they want to know our deepest secrets? Perhaps our sexual fantasies? First I'd note that the therapist is not obliged to respond if it feels unsafe or unhelpful. Beyond that, I suppose these deeply invasive types of questions *are* possible, but only if the patient really wants to challenge the therapeutic relationship they've built. And that, too, is valuable information.

Yes, I felt strongly Gene had gifted me something useful, a way to prompt the self-disclosure process I've been exploring, focused on areas of my life that would be of interest to particular patients. It seemed probable this would quickly bring to the forefront areas that challenged them. I also liked how this tool might give patients a greater sense of agency. I looked forward to exploring further when the right opportunities arose.

CHAPTER 15

Let's Switch Roles

I n the weeks following my meeting with Gene, I experimented several times with the role reversal strategy, which she had inadvertently gifted me. In each case I employed the tactic with a patient who was struggling to open up, who kept our discussion on a surface level and dared not risk revealing their inner selves. I would suggest some variation on the idea that we should switch places for a bit and that they should ask me questions. I encouraged them to ask anything they desired and promised to answer as truthfully as I could. Each time, giving them this power seemed to move us toward greater intimacy and helped them open up. Alara was one of these early encounters.

Alara's email had given me some basic information. She was a forty-year-old Turkish woman, living in Istanbul with her husband and three children, twin twelve-year-old sons and a two-year-old daughter. As a child her family had been moderately wealthy, enough so that she had been educated at private schools and spoke excellent English. Unfortunately her father's import-export business had recently collapsed, and he had lost most of his wealth trying to save it. Alara and her sisters now supported her parents.

Alara did not wait for me to begin our session and right away said, "I imagine that your first question must be 'Why have you asked to see me?'"

"You're entirely correct. That is generally my opening question."

"And my answer is that I have been in COVID lockdown for a year, and it is driving me crazy."

"Tell me what's happening for you," I said.

"I am lonely and confined. The same isolated life day after day after day. But, no, that is not the issue. It is not the day. It is the night. We have a two-year-old daughter who sleeps in our bed. She is a wiggler, and my husband and I get very little rest. Our apartment has three small bedrooms. What was the baby's bedroom is now packed full of computer equipment, where my husband works twelve hours a day. He is in tech and now, like everyone else, works from home. Our two boys and their toys and clothes fill the second room. So the only place for our two-year-old is in our bed."

"That doesn't leave much room for you, Alara," I said.

"Mmmm," she responded, as if she barely heard me.

"And no privacy for you and your husband."

"Mmmm. My daughter is restless and sleeps poorly," she continued.

Through all of this she never looked at me. Rather she stared off to the side, as if watching something over my shoulder. I asked her to describe a typical night. She told me that she often takes her crying daughter onto the balcony outside the bedroom, and she thinks about jumping into the traffic below and killing herself. She said this with a strange, almost sweet smile on her face, still looking off to the side. I didn't know what to make of it, a patient talking so calmly about suicide. Generally there is at least some discomfort at bringing up the subject—often a sense of shame or even embarrassment.

"Can you tell me more about these thoughts of suicide?" I asked, trying to gauge how serious this was.

"It is nothing new," she said, as if it weren't important.

"Do you ever make plans?"

"I would not actually do it."

"But the thought is there."

"Mmmm."

I waited, and after a minute she continued.

"This is just a passing thought. Like noticing the weather."

"And what are the patterns of the weather?"

"Sometimes clear. Sometimes much darker."

"And when it is darker . . . ?"

I waited again. She gave a soft smile. I had the feeling she was primarily impressing on me that the situation was painful but that she was used to it. Sadness, but not desperation. When it was clear she wasn't going to say anything further, I made a mental note to come back to this. Then I pivoted and asked about her inability to sleep, as sleep is so closely tied to so many aspects of how we feel.

"It has been happening for a long time," she told me. "It's nothing new."

"Have you spoken to your doctor about your lack of sleep? Or perhaps a therapist?"

Alara stared back at me with an oddly guileless look on her face, as though neither thought had ever occurred to her. Again I didn't know what to make of her. Some of her responses were so quick and clear, but others seemed slow and disconnected, as if her mind had floated off elsewhere. Was she stoned? Or somehow delayed in her comprehension?

I asked again about her experience with therapy, and she responded casually that one of her twin sons had been seeing a psychologist for two years. I was about to suggest that she might benefit from ongoing therapy, given her suicidal thoughts, when she spontaneously recounted a vague dream she had the night before involving her grandmother, who had died seven years ago and who had spent her entire life taking care of her children and grandchildren. I asked for more details, but Alara didn't offer any. I asked what feelings the dream had evoked for her. No response. I wondered aloud if she herself were afraid of spending her life caring for others. Again no response.

I was perplexed. She kept offering bits of information about her experience and her serious concerns, but only brief slivers, with no curiosity about connecting them. Then she'd fall back into an almost childlike naivete. Somehow I had to get her to go deeper, to shake off whatever was holding her back. This was when, in an effort to coax her engaged adult self out of hiding, I thought about reversing roles.

"Alara, I've been the one asking questions. I'd like to suggest that we try something different. Let's you and I switch roles for a few minutes. What questions do you have for me? I give you my word I will respond to any question you ask. And the deeper, the more personal, the better."

I expected her to be shocked or puzzled. To my surprise, she looked directly at me for the first time, and spoke confidently. "I am interested in how you became interested in the relationship between philosophy and psychology."

Now I was the one who was shocked. Given the detached

way she had been speaking, I had not expected such a cerebral question. So as not to betray my surprise, I rushed to answer. "Good question, Alara. I grew up in a poor neighborhood in Washington, DC, that wasn't very safe. I spent a great deal of my childhood alone, reading in the library or at home, and I've never stopped reading. Books, particularly ones with strong, juicy plots, were my friends, and my escape, I suppose, from a hard reality. Then I went into medicine, not because I was truly passionate about it but by necessity. My parents were immigrant Russian Jews with no education. For me and others like me, it seemed like there were only two possible ways to gain respect and live a good life: you became a doctor or you became a lawyer. I chose the former, which meant years of studying science. I found it interesting sometimes. But really I craved literature. I craved stories! So after years of memorizing anatomic structures and differential diagnoses, it seemed the closest I could come to literature in medicine was the field of psychiatry."

"Yes, people, our minds, and our problems. That makes sense!" Alara seemed enlivened, alert. "Then what?"

"Well, when I was doing my residency in psychiatry I read a new book called *Existence* by a therapist named Rollo May. It wasn't about diagnosis or pharmacology, the things I mostly encountered in my training, but rather about deep ideas like where people find value, or if one person's sensory experiences are the same as another's, things like that. It helped me imagine that philosophy could play a major role in psychotherapy. I immediately decided to obtain an education in philosophy, and I began taking night courses at Johns Hopkins University."

"So, this Rollo May was your teacher?"

"Not officially. But I learned a lot from his books. Then, a few years later when I was leading a therapy group for patients with untreatable cancers, I became extremely anxious about death. I met Rollo for the first time and began therapy as his patient. That treatment, and that connection with him, was very helpful to me."

As we continued, Alara seemed to mature in front of my eyes. She started asking questions about my therapy with Rollo. How did he think about death? Did he cure me of my anxiety? What did I learn from him? Where do people find meaning? Her transformation seemed miraculous. Gone was the naive woman with the fixed childlike smile on her face. In her place was an energetic young woman, eager for engagement and dialogue. I told her how surprised and pleased I was to see this change come over her. I asked what had caused this change and why she had been so remote earlier.

"This is the real me," she said after some hesitation. "But there are some personal things that are very difficult to discuss. Things that involve my husband and which, if made public, would wound him deeply."

"As a therapist, I would never reveal anything that would cause pain to you or to him."

"But you are more than a therapist. You are a writer."

Ah! A revelation. Suddenly the contrast between engaged Alara and distant Alara became clearer.

"Yes," I responded, "I'm so glad you're speaking so openly. Please know that I am a therapist before I am a writer, and I have vowed that I would never ever write anything that would injure my patients. If I write anything, I always thoroughly disguise the patient's identity. And I always seek explicit permission to publish."

Alara looked into my eyes for a few moments, nodded, and said, "My husband is very fragile. He has a great fear of death. Maybe it is similar to you. You said you saw Rollo May because of your fear about death. My husband's father died when he was seven years old, and he and his mother are still grieving deeply for him. Whenever his mother visits, they go into a corner and talk and talk and weep about his father."

"But he must have died thirty years ago—"

"Thirty-six," Alara interrupted. "My husband simply will not talk about his father's death, or death in general."

"How difficult. How disabling."

"The very mention of death shuts him down completely. Imagine, my sons find a dead bird, and I can say nothing about it if their father is nearby. At best I try to explain in whispers."

"This must disrupt your life considerably."

"Very much. It is the source of my despair. That, and the lack of sleep."

I tried to imagine how hard it would be to live in this world where death exists, for all of us, without being able to mention it. So much energy, so much life, would be exhausted in avoidance.

"I've rarely heard such an extreme case," I said. "Please urge your husband to see a good therapist to help him with this."

"I have done that many times, but he refuses very strongly."

"Because?"

"He won't say. But I'm sure it's fear of being made to confront death."

"Hmmm. What if you tell him that you want to be in couples therapy? That would help the two of you, and it may be a way of sneaking in some therapy that could help him individually."

"What do you mean?"

"A stealth project of sorts. You can talk about other issues in your relationship, the sleep problem, challenges with your family, whatever feels useful. Then, eventually, you can bring up ways your husband's death anxiety impacts you. A good therapist will be able to tease this out and work with it."

She nodded, intrigued but wary.

"And if he resists the suggestion of couples therapy at first, you might share with him that you are having suicidal thoughts, and that you need him to work on this with you. That might allow him to feel he is not giving up control but rather doing something for your sake."

"That would shake him up," she reflected. "He might be willing."

I said I would ask a Turkish colleague for referrals in Istanbul.

"I have one last question, Dr. Yalom," Alara said. "I read your last book about your wife's death, and I would like to ask about how you are doing now in your grief. Is it okay to ask you something so . . . so personal?"

"I like your being so personal. It's the way I want you and your husband to be. Let me share that I'm still in grief, and life isn't as much fun anymore. I'm not surprised by this. I've known Marilyn and loved her since I was fourteen years old and I knew I would be in grief for a long, long time. I, too, think about death a lot these days. Her death, and my own. It no longer overwhelms me. I've lived a good life, quite fully. Nonetheless, at night I enjoy watching happy films. This week I've really been cheered up by the old film *Lili* with Leslie Caron."

"Thank you for being so open, Dr. Yalom. It helps. And let me offer you the gift of *An American in Paris*. Leslie Caron is in that one, too. It has excellent dance scenes."

Four weeks later Alara sent me an email saying that her husband had, very reluctantly, agreed to at least explore couples therapy. Her message had another gift for me, lines that read:

*. . . I've realized that the most important effect of our meet-
ing came from you being so connected and present from the
very first moment, with me—a complete stranger. I rarely
experience this in everyday life. I don't know if anyone does.
Thank you.*

How lovely to have Alara remind me of my own professional
mantra, that "it is the relationship that heals." That is to say, a
patient's growth and change comes as a result of experiences
in the context of a close, safe bond with their therapist more
than from any particular intervention, diagnosis, or medication. In several of these stories I have mentioned the need to
build this trusting connection as essential for here-and-now
work. But I would go further and say that *whatever* approach
one has to therapy, from short-term solution-focused therapy
to cognitive behavioral therapy to long-term psychodynamic
analysis, building a strong trusting positive relationship with
one's patients is critical. I was glad to see this proven again in
my sessions with Alara.

Clearly this relationship building in a onetime session is
particularly challenging. But if I am to take my own mantra seriously, and believe that the relationship is indeed the
mechanism of healing, then in these single hours I must focus
great attention on how to build those relationships quickly.
Sharing of oneself—one's vulnerability, one's compassion,
one's humanity—and encouraging the patient to do the same
may not be the only way to achieve this, but it certainly is
what works best for me.

To have Alara reflect that so clearly was lovely. Revealing
parts of my history was immensely helpful in getting Alara to
quickly move past her initial reluctance to open up. And the
role-reversal technique proved effective in engaging her. But I

can imagine that many therapists, especially young ones, may find this approach uncomfortable. It requires a great degree of openness. Fortunately I am at a stage of my life, its last sliver, in which I no longer feel (much) need to keep things secret or to protect myself (much) from the opinions of others. This general imperviousness to outside opinion allows me to explore this method easily. So let me continue exploring. My hope is that this investigation will be helpful to young therapists in determining to what degree this strategy is useful.

CHAPTER 16

My Worst Nightmare

The experiments with radical self-disclosure in these chapters are not entirely new. Since the beginning of my career, I have embraced transparency in terms of my feelings about my patients, elicited their honest feelings about me, and looked together at what is going on between us in real time. The short adventures of these very direct single consultations have pushed this core idea further: in tightening the time frame I've forced myself to push harder and to reveal more, faster. Thus far I have been amazed at the powerful results.

And yet one must be careful. The wrong kinds of self-revelation can be harmful. Most patients won't be helped by a therapist preening about their own successes or sharing thoughts that simply aren't relevant to the patient's problems. List these blunders as "not helpful," I suppose. But there are other mistakes one might make—if one were, say, a forgetful nearly ninety-year-old man—that are far, far worse.

One sunny day in May, over a year into COVID, I had a

particularly challenging session with a woman named Rose. Afterward I did what I always do: I reviewed my handwritten notes, then dictated a summary into my iPhone and emailed it to myself to store in her file on my computer.

This is one of the most disappointing consultations I've done! Rose is 35, with a 12-year-old daughter. She and her husband divorced 11 years ago, and she remains dependent on him financially through alimony and child support. She hopes to be entirely self-supporting, and is currently in her final year of a PhD program in clinical psychology.

She was extremely vague throughout our conversation, and I could not understand much of what she said. Sentences like fleecy clouds passed through her lips, ungraspable, wafting lazily across the room. I had trouble understanding what she was experiencing. I simply could not get her to clarify what she wanted to work on.

I tried to address this several times by moving into the here and now, which almost always clarifies the encounter. Not today. Each time Rose stared blankly at me.

Toward the end of our hour together, Rose began to weep and wiped her eyes with Kleenex. I asked, as I often do at such times, "If those tears could speak, what would they say?" This question is a silver bullet! It rarely fails to get things going. But it totally flopped, and Rose looked mystified, as if I were speaking Mandarin or Aramaic.

Several times I interrupted and told her that I was puzzled by her comments. "Please, can you be clearer?" I asked, but always without effect. I was left frustrated at not being able to connect with her or offer any help. The vagueness persisted, and at the end of our session I knew little about Rose. Worse, I am sure she received little of value from me.

I consider this the least successful of these single-session consultations!

Imagine my shock when, a few hours later, she emailed that summary back to me, accompanied by the following:

Dr. Yalom,
I have a feeling that these are your personal notes which you had certainly not intended to send to me. But you did, so I will respond. I've been in tears continually after reading that our meeting was your least satisfying consultation ever. I'm shocked. I've encountered criticism from other people, but I had hoped that things would be different with you.
   In our session I felt you were asking me to give you something that I don't know how to give. I am not always able to identify, much less say, exactly what I am feeling in the moment, and time pressure makes it even harder. And you were very, very persistent.
   I've been working on being aware and authentic. Yoga and meditation help. But then sometimes, with some people, all my gains fly out the window. Sometimes I find the words later, but in the moment I am unable to grasp them. There are many people I can be open with. Why couldn't I be open with you? I don't yet understand. Now I just feel foolish for making the attempt and I can't stop crying.

My god, what had I done!? This was undoubtedly one of the worst blunders I'd ever made with a patient. Not only had I not helped her, I had sent her into despair. Feeling queasy and wanting desperately to fix the damage I'd caused, I immediately responded with profuse apologies and deep embarrassment, explaining that the notes were for my eyes only. I asked if she would please let me offer her another session free of charge, and that perhaps we could forge a better connection. I thought she might just as well prefer that I take a long walk off the proverbially short pier, but I offered nonetheless.

Guilt quickly enveloped me, and I found I could barely move from my office desk. I perseverated for a few minutes about the mechanics of the incident, how I must have received my own email and with clumsy fingers somehow forwarded it on to her. I could not remember actually doing this, which was another disconcerting indication of memory loss, but I must have. She had received it and was now suffering pain that I had carelessly inflicted. I thought to get up and walk back up the path to the house, feeling that perhaps being outside in the California sun would help. But I found myself glued to my seat. Never, not in sixty-five years of practicing, have I ever sent a patient my negative feelings about a session. In fact, I've never heard of *any* therapist making such a catastrophic blunder! A voice in the back of my mind squeaked that this was the sign I'd been dreading, the sign that it was time to hang it all up.

Then, fortunately, the familiar ping of an email arriving, Rose granting me a reprieve. Yes, she would like to try another meeting. But not until her finals were over, as she couldn't risk the stress of more emotional turmoil before her exams.

We planned to meet again ten days later. I was anxious, very anxious. I hadn't felt this nervous about a patient in decades, possibly not since I was a young intern awaiting the harsh critique of the attending psychiatrists at Mount Sinai. I worked to calm myself. I took several deep breaths and prepared to focus on her needs, not my anxiety.

Ordinarily I go into a session intending to help in any possible way I can. Today the goal was different: simply to undo the damage I had wrought. I began as soon as her face appeared.

"Rose, I want to offer my apologies. I'm so sorry for having upset you. That's the last thing I wanted to do."

"Then why did you write it?" she asked, a bit sternly.

"What you saw were my personal notes of the session, to remind me of how *I* felt. It was only meant for me. I feel very stupid, awful, about you seeing that. I do a lot of work assessing my own feelings with my patients, and I felt I hadn't helped you very much."

"Imagine how *I* felt."

"I can only imagine you must have felt betrayed."

"Betrayed. Yes, that's the correct word. The perfect word."

"Please keep in mind, Rose, it was a blunder. It was a letter from myself to myself reminding me of the feelings I had."

"Yes, your memory is poor, I know. You warned me at the outset. Still, I shouldn't have to suffer because of that."

If I had harbored any thought of escaping by blaming my failing brain, Rose made it clear that path wasn't open. On the plus side, she was definitely engaged now, and that gave me something to work with.

"Can you share more about your reaction to my note?"

Unlike our previous session, she had no trouble responding.

"Blackness! Despair! The depression I had reading that note after our session was the worst I've experienced since getting divorced. The main reason I have slogged through this PhD program is that I never want to be dependent on a man again. Yet, here I am, with a powerful man attacking me."

It began to dawn on me that her vagueness and avoidance in our previous session came from a place of fear. She had been hurt before and was still under the power of her ex-husband, who controlled her finances. Opening up to me could be frightening. It would be devastating if, for instance, she showed me her deepest concerns, her vulnerabilities, and rather than tend them lovingly, I rejected her in some way as a result. No wonder she had been unable to participate. I felt a bit slow and stupid. I tried to modulate my voice and speak more gently.

"Rose, what was most striking to me in our first session was your reluctance to engage me in the here and now. On several occasions I asked about how you and I were doing in the session or what you were feeling toward me, and *that's* when you really froze up. I was confused about this, but now I'm realizing that you must have been very frightened of me. After all, I did put a lot of pressure on you by asking you about what was happening between us."

"That's part of it, your persistence," Rose quickly replied. "Add in that your group therapy book is the main text for one of my classes, we're reading your inpatient group book in another, and *Love's Executioner* is what got me interested in being a therapist to begin with. Having a session with you was something I really, really wanted to do. But honestly, I was not prepared for an interrogation."

Yikes! I felt faint. In our first session she had mentioned her studies, but somehow it hadn't clicked. *Why didn't she remind me of this?* I thought. *Why didn't she tell me she's studying my textbooks?* The answer from within appeared instantly: *BECAUSE SHE IS TERRIFIED OF YOU, YOU JERK!*

"Rose," I said, "suddenly the mystery is unraveling. It's not that you're unable to engage; it's that you're extremely frightened of me! Your image of *Dr. Irvin Yalom* must have loomed huge in your imagination."

Rose looked at me for a long time.

"Am I right? Is the mystery unraveling?"

Rose nodded. "I agree. Yes, entirely. Talking with the author of our textbooks, whom my teachers admire so much, was scary. Too scary to even say it was scary."

"Something is changing now. I think we're making progress," I said. "Now that I understand how difficult it is for you to answer my very persistent questioning, I have a suggestion. Let's try something else, okay? You can be the . . . interrogator. You ask me some questions."

Rose looked at me quizzically.

"I'm entirely serious, Rose. Give it a try. I promise to answer any question you ask."

Rose closed her eyes for a few moments and then took the plunge. She asked me, as several patients have done, how I was coping with my wife's death, and I began to tell her, as I have told many others, how inseparable Marilyn and I had been since adolescence, how my prospects for happiness and health were poor now, how seeing my children helped, when she cut me off.

"Thank you, Irv. But let me be more clear, less 'fleecy.' When I asked how are you coping with it, I was really wondering what are you doing to deal with the grief? How do you get through your days?"

"Ah. No one has asked me that. I—"

I had to pause for a moment to consider this. This felt a little tender for me, and I noted an impulse to protect myself by revealing less. I took this reluctance as a sign to be as transparent as I could.

"Thank you for asking a challenging question, Rose. Mostly I have been writing. In her last months, Marilyn wanted the two of us to write a book together about her illness and death. We wrote alternating chapters about her last months, and after she died I wrote the second half. We decided to call it *A*

Matter of Death and Life—that is, Marilyn's death and my life after. Working on that book kept me busy enough to be a bit distracted. And because it was about her death, I guess it gave me the familiar container of writing to contemplate the most unfamiliar and frightening experience. I dreaded finishing the book, but eventually I had to turn it over to my editor. Now I'm consulting with people like you, which gives me great pleasure. And I'm writing about some of these encounters. Otherwise, to be completely honest with you, Rose, my days are lonely and rather bleak."

I stopped, and we sat in silence for a few poignant moments.

"Now let me ask you a question, Rose, a here-and-now question. How did you feel about what I just told you?"

"Touched. I feel . . . I don't know how to put it. Maybe a bit honored that you would trust me in that way, that you would be so open. I'm not sure I deserve it."

"Why?"

"Well, you gave me so much more than I gave you."

Something had changed drastically between us, and I told her so. "In our first, disastrous consultation, when I asked about how you and I were doing, you froze up. I kept badgering you with questions—so very persistently, as you put it—and I concluded that you were unable to discuss the immediate present, unable to handle intimacy, for whatever reason. But I was completely mistaken. What really happened was that you were extremely frightened of me, too frightened even to tell me you were frightened."

"Yes. I was terrified. And you made a mistake. It's surprising that you are willing to admit that. A good lesson. Thank you."

"Learning to admit our errors *is* a good lesson. And let me admit something else, Rose. I'm truly embarrassed to say this, but today, before you mentioned the textbooks, I had forgotten you were studying clinical psychology. Too much data for my old brain."

"Forgotten? What is it about me that causes you to forget?"

"That is a great response for a therapist looking at the space between people! But trust me, Rose, in this case the problem is entirely on my end. I am getting *seriously* old—I'll be ninety next month—and my memory is really failing me. I've been seeing a new patient in consultation every single day, probably as much to distract myself from dark thoughts of my impending mortality as to help others. Maybe it's too much, too many to keep track of."

She did not contradict this. I sat, feeling miserable for a moment, until Rose spoke up with sudden enthusiasm.

"Oh yeah! I've got one more question! This whole mess started because you mistakenly mailed me your private notes, right?"

I felt a wave of anxiety, fearing she was going to dig further into my failure. I nodded for her to continue.

"You said you dictated your notes of our consultation onto your iPhone. I'm curious about that. Tell me, why did you email that to yourself? I don't get it."

"Well, the dictated note is on my iPhone, and I wanted to send it to my computer, where I keep all my records. There is no good way of dictating directly onto my computer, because the software doesn't work very well. It seems to keep cutting me off. So, I hit upon the clever idea of emailing the iPhone notes to myself and saving them on my computer. I just email to myself and, presto, problem solved."

Rose burst out laughing.

"What's happening, Rose? Tell me, what's making you laugh? What's so funny?"

"I'd prefer to show rather than to tell. And to do that, we

have to end this Zoom call and continue by phone. Here's my number." She rattled it off and I wrote it down.

"So, Irv, here's what to do. Please phone me as soon as you end this Zoom session, but keep your computer on and in front of you."

I followed her directions and dialed her phone number.

"Hi," she answered. "Now I'm going to answer your question by giving you some clear and simple directions that even an old man with a bad memory should be able to follow. I want you to look at the row of icons, probably on the side of the screen. Got it?"

"Got it. I see the long row on the left side of my screen. Now what?"

"On my computer, the top icon shows the Finder. It's a smiling face—both in profile and straight on. It's blue and white."

"Mine, too. Blue and white face. I see it."

"Good. Now go down the row and you'll see an icon with a yellow band on the top that says 'Notes' when you put the cursor on it. Now click on it."

"I see it and I'm clicking on it."

"What do you see?"

"Good lord! I see a list of names—dozens of them."

"They are in order according to date. Go down to November twelfth, the date of our first meeting, and tell me what you see."

"I see your name. And, wait, there is the summary of our session—that dreadful summary. How did this get here?"

"What do you think?"

"I think I'm slow and, possibly, a bit stupid. Do you mean to tell me that every time I dictate on 'Notes' on my iPhone, it automatically goes to my computer?"

"Every time," said Rose, who was having difficulty contain-
ing her laughter.

"So all these months when I've been sending summaries to
my computer, they were, in fact, already there? And my brilliant, clever, deeply original idea of emailing myself is entirely
ludicrous?"

"Glad to be of help."

"Hmm, so this guy, Yalom, who wrote the textbook you use,
who is esteemed by your teachers and who intimidates you,
can sometimes be a bit of a bonehead?"

"And *he* keeps on teaching me."

"How so?"

"Well, he's up front and totally open with what he doesn't
know. I respect that."

"Remember when I said I am writing about some of these
consultations? I'm focusing on the useful lessons I'm learning and, of course, the most interesting encounters. Despite
my embarrassment—or maybe because of it—I'm feeling that
there might be a good story arising from our meeting."

"You mean you might write a story about us? Oh, I hope
you will!"

"One thing I can promise," I said, "is that if I *do* write our
story, I'll ask for your permission, and I'll make sure I send it
to the right person!"

Earlier, when this comedy of errors began, I wrote that I had
never even heard of a therapist accidentally sharing their confi-
dential notes with a patient. Apparently my memory of my own
work is slipping away just like everything else. On first reading
this, my collaborator, Ben, pointed out that twenty-five years
ago I wrote a story as part of the collection *Momma and the
Meaning of Life* called "Double Exposure" that hinges on my

fictional alter ego, Ernest Lash, accidentally sending a patient, Linda, home with an audio recording of his notes about her. Hearing his very blunt and harsh thoughts, Linda is enormously upset. But rather than reveal the error, as Rose did for me, she proceeds to torture Ernest for several months, using many of his unkind descriptions of her against him—that she bores him with her repetitious complaints, that she is vulgar and grasping for money. She even weaponizes his sexual feelings toward her, information she knows full well from the accidental recording. She is sharp and scolding, and definitely makes Lash pay the price for his blunder. In retrospect, I wonder if my great anxiety before my second session with Rose was bolstered by a deep-seated memory of this, a subconscious fear that I would be taken to task in the same scathing way that Ernest was, all of which would be entirely my fault.

What is similar between "Double Exposure" and this session with Rose is that in both cases the accidental revelations eventually lead to more open and healing relationships between the patient and therapist. I'm not such a Pollyanna to believe this will always be the case, and there are certainly better ways to develop intimacy than to pass on one's private uncensored notes. But therapists make mistakes all the time. If one is able and willing to address them with transparency and humility, it often presents an opportunity for growth and transformation, whether you are at the beginning of your career or the very tail end.

CHAPTER 17

Memory, Memory, Where Art Thou?

I f one is willing to donate a substantial amount of money to the city of Palo Alto, California, one is permitted to place a memorial plaque to a loved one on one of the benches in Bol Park, down the hill from my home. When Marilyn died, I selected a bench set between oak and walnut trees and commissioned this plaque.

> **MARILYN YALOM**
> SCHOLAR, AUTHOR,
> TEACHER, FEMINIST, AND
> MASTER CHUTNEY CHEF.
>
> SHE IS MUCH MISSED
> BY HER FOUR CHILDREN:
> EVE, REID, VICTOR, AND BEN.
> AND BY IRV, HER HUSBAND
> OF SIXTY-FIVE YEARS:
> A LONG MARRIAGE BUT
> NOT NEARLY LONG ENOUGH

Almost every day around 5:00 p.m. I push my walker on a twenty-minute stroll to Marilyn's bench. Once there, I speak to Marilyn's spirit, the one in my mind, recounting my day to her and reiterating how much I love and miss her. She was a great walker, and our walks together were much longer. But the years have sapped my energy and stolen certain capacities, like my balance, so now I move slowly and a bit unevenly, pushing my walker in front of me, drawn to her bench but no farther.

Neighbors who walk in the park are used to seeing me here, and occasionally fans leave me notes pinned to the bench. One day a therapist from the Middle East was waiting for me on the bench and brought me a present—a sizable package of halvah. She claimed that somewhere in one of my books she had read that as a child I had loved halvah, and she wished to offer me some as a way of thanking me for the books I had written. Of course I have no memory of writing that, but the halvah was delicious, and this idea provides a little intrigue for my daily stroll—what else might be waiting for me that I once mentioned enjoying? A science fiction novel? A Joe DiMaggio rookie card? A corned beef sandwich?

Several days after my ninetieth birthday, I was sitting on the bench and communing with Marilyn when an enjoyable memory surfaced. For years I used to ride my bike in the afternoons, getting some exercise after sedentary hours writing and seeing patients. I remembered the feeling of movement, of wheels turning under me and gentle wind in my face. Across the park I could see the sandy playground where my children spent sunny afternoons, and where grandchildren and even great-grandchildren still play when visiting. From some corner of my mind another memory emerged: I was pulling a rubbery monster mask over my head, a mask with fangs, bright blood spatters, and long matted hair. Then I was riding my bike past the playground, making cartoon screeching sounds to entertain, or perhaps frighten, the kids. Could I have done such a thing? I'll have to ask Eve.

I was lost in this reverie when an elderly woman stopped near the bench and greeted me warmly.

"Hi, Irv," she said with a smile. "I'm Debbie, just in case you've forgotten. We haven't seen each other in years and for me, at least, matching names to faces seems to get harder and harder. May I sit? There is something I very much want to ask you."

"Of course, Debbie," I responded, while wondering who *was* this woman?

After joining me on the bench, she smiled, looked me up and down, and began, "I've had some bad news and need some help. You're the only therapist I feel I can rely on, and I miss your presence in my life. I stopped by your old house up the street to say hello and to ask for an appointment with you. The folks living there now told me you had moved to the next block many years ago. They also said I might find you at this bench and, well, here you are."

She was very familiar—her voice, her face—yet I could not place her. How frustrating. She was perhaps ten to fifteen years younger than me, but then pretty much everyone was younger than me at this point, so that wasn't a great deal of help. She must have been a patient of mine long ago, I thought, but I could not recall a single detail of our past connection.

Ah memory! Every day I received some further reminder that it continued to flake away. I was so embarrassed by this that I generally tried to hide it from others as much as possible.

One of my worst fears was that someone in an official capacity would tell me I was no longer fit to offer therapy. Hence,
I rarely acknowledged my memory failure. Instead, I would
fall back on my old poker-playing skills and bluff to buy time.
Generally, after a few minutes of conversation, some stalks
of memory would emerge and soon everything would come
flooding back. With that in mind, I turned to her, determined
to draw out more information until something crystallized.

"Tell me, Debbie, what's happened?"

"Well, to sum up quickly, I need some help. Two weeks ago,
a lifelong friend died."

"I'm so sorry to hear it."

"It gets more complicated. We had a serious falling-out just
days before. My fault, really. She's been my closest friend for
many years and I'm having enormous difficulty dealing with
her death. I want very much to have a session with you. I know
that we haven't met for decades but I trust you, Irv, and I'd be
so grateful if you'd schedule me for an appointment as soon
as possible."

I told her that I was no longer seeing patients for ongoing
therapy but that I'd be happy to meet for a consultation. "Let
me look at my schedule when I return home, and I'll send you
some possible times. Could you write down your email for
me?" She quickly opened her purse, jotted her email address
on a notepad, tore it off, and handed it to me.

"Great, Irv. And include your fee in your email. I imagine it's
gone up since we last met. Mine sure has. All my peers charge
at least two hundred dollars per session, and psychiatrists like
you, four hundred dollars minimum. Silicon Valley certainly
changed everything. Remember when this was a quiet college
town?" She smiled, then turned and strolled off.

I looked at the note she'd handed me. Just an email address.

Why hadn't I asked her to write more? A last name sure would
have helped. Ah well. As I slowly returned home with the
assistance of my trusty walker, I kept sifting through the information I had. She called me "Irv" and she seemed to have
known me well, if long ago. She was a therapist, probably a
clinical psychologist, and clearly not a psychiatrist. And she
had been my patient at some point. I kept sifting through my
brain, but I could not recall treating her.

By the time I arrived home, I'd narrowed the era down to
the mid- to late seventies and guessed that she was a therapist
who worked in the Stanford outpatient clinic, which I had run
for many years. This seemed close, but it couldn't be entirely
correct because I would never have treated someone with
whom I worked regularly. I put the question on a back burner
and figured I would have to wait for our upcoming session to
discover the truth.

I emailed her a time the following week for our appointment and told her that I would send a Zoom invitation shortly
before our meeting.

She emailed back immediately. "Irv, I recently got my two
vaccinations and the pandemic is waning. I'd so much prefer
to meet with you in person—like in the good old days when
we were both young."

This happened during that brief window in time, the summer of 2021, when it seemed the world was opening back up.
Vaccinations made it feel like even we fragile old folks might
be safe from COVID, and the next wave of aggressive virus
variants hadn't yet hit. I had not seen a live patient in my office
in well over a year. In fact, I had rarely seen live humans in the
flesh other than my children and a few friends. But the timing
was right, and I, too, had been twice vaccinated. I agreed to
a face-to-face meeting and added that I looked forward to it.

A few days later we met in my office. For the first half of our session we focused on her friend Jill's death and Debbie's strong sense of guilt about the argument they'd had. Jill's husband had advanced dementia, and Jill had been having an affair with her neighbor, who was married. Debbie had disapproved intensely of the affair, so much so that these two best friends had not talked in weeks. Then Jill died of a heart attack and Debbie was overcome with grief and regret about her judgmental behavior. I made careful notes of her story, while simultaneously searching for any further clues of just who Debbie was to me and who I was to her. Nothing was coming to me yet.

Together we looked at her overpowering sense of guilt, and I impressed upon her that she was not responsible for Jill's heart attack, nor her choices in romantic partners. I inquired about Debbie's intense response to Jill's affair. Why had this upset her so much? Was it a moral judgment? Or perhaps she had her own experience with infidelity that had colored her feelings? We talked through several possibilities, with Debbie engaged, curious, and also at a bit of a loss to explain her powerful reaction.

"I just don't know for sure," she said. "It's times like these that I really miss our group. I miss it so much!"

Our group?! There was a possible clue.

But what group was she referring to? Much of my early work was as a group therapist, and my book *The Theory and Practice of Group Therapy* is what had really made my name in the field. In the sixties and seventies I led so many therapy groups, eager to distill what made them so effective, eager to help people help each other, constantly fascinated by the dynamics and experimenting with the structure. I led long-term groups through the Stanford outpatient clinic, short-term groups at the inpatient clinic, as well as cancer patient groups, bereavement groups, general process groups. So many. Which group was she talking about?

And why *our* group? She was a therapist, so perhaps we had co-led a group, something I often did with colleagues. I just couldn't remember. I was flooded with frustration. Imagine working closely with someone, possibly for years, and then simply not being able to recognize them. Imagine *knowing you know them*, but not being able to put the pieces together in your mind.

After frustration came a wave of shame. Admitting my decline has been very hard, even with people I encounter only once over Zoom. But here, in person, with Debbie, who clearly had a much closer relationship with me, and with the me at the peak of my capacities, when I was truly making discoveries and having an impact—just then the truth that I couldn't even remember her felt too painful to reveal. At the same time I did not want to hurt her by telling her I did not recall *our* group, which seemed so very important to her. Perhaps these were only rationalizations, excuses to avoid disclosing my decline. Whatever the case, avoid I did. I pushed forward hoping that she would say something that would crack open the floodgates of memory.

"Tell me more about our group," I suggested.

"Irv, I don't recall having said this to you, but you *must* have known that our group was incredibly important to me. It was the highlight of my week for several years. I'll always be grateful to you, and the other members, for that experience. Truly." She paused and reached for a tissue. "Last week when I went to your old house, I took a long, nostalgic look at the room over the garage where we met for all those years. Your neighbor told me that there is an elderly couple living there now."

Our old house. A room over the garage. All those years.

Boom! A memory exploded in my mind, and then several more. People sitting on a U-shaped sofa, mottled brown carpet beneath our feet, dappled sunlight streaming through windows. I began to remember! It was a very particular group that met in the writing studio I'd built at my home, a space apart from the official aegis of the university. It was made up not of psychiatric patients but of fellow therapists. This made it quite unusual but also necessary, as therapists are often reluctant to be in a group with non-therapists because of the imbalance in knowledge of the process. It was a structure I'd put in place to establish a setting where members could experience the great interpersonal learning of being inside the group therapy process, while also feeling they were among peers, all astute at looking at the emotions and impulses that came up in the room as they related to one another.

Debbie's nostalgia made perfect sense. The group had been very important to me, too: it was a major event of my week for years. We met every Thursday evening in that studio, which was built on the second floor, nestled among the branches of several large oak trees. It was warm, well lit, and forever a bit dusty. The level of connection that I felt for the members was unusually deep. I suspect this was in part because we were all professionals with similar interests, and in part because of the long duration of the group. It continued for many years, with members occasionally leaving as they landed positions elsewhere or simply moved on with their lives, and new members joining when spots opened up.

Those early years at Stanford were remarkable. The time was full of innovation and excitement. I arrived just as the university was developing a new psychiatry department. The chair, David Hamburg, hired a group of young professors at the same time and gave each a specific assignment—head of student health services, head of the inpatient hospital program, head of outpatient services. In a stroke of cosmic good luck, I was the only one left unassigned. When I asked what my responsibilities would be, Dr. Hamburg told me that he'd been impressed by the articles I'd written and that it was my job to continue thinking, exploring, writing. What a glorious charter! And so I set about leading therapy groups, distilling their power into core ideas, and experimenting with different nuances of therapy. I also spent a lot of time learning about other currents in the field, such as the imaginative and groundbreaking work that was happening nearby at the Mental Research Institute, where radically new approaches to therapy focused on families and couples were being developed. It was a rich, heady time to be a psychiatrist tasked with exploring and advancing the field!

The group that Debbie brought me back to was one of those exciting explorations. I felt some chagrin that I had forgotten that particular group. Now that I'd identified it, none of the group members reappeared in my mind, even though I *knew* these had been some of the most profound relationships in my life for a long period. It was a quandary. My ego reared up as well, and I did not want her to know just how much I, once the respected leader, had been reduced. And yet I yearned to hear more, to access her memories, which might replenish mine.

"Tell me of any news you have about the members," I ventured, treading carefully.

"Well. I attended Gloria's wedding last year. She seemed very happy."

Gloria. Gloria? Nope, nothing.

"News about any of the others?" I asked.

"Some bad news. Paul died recently, cancer. And Bertha, too, about ten years ago."

"Oh yes," I said. Bertha's face came to mind, round, with a crooked smile. She was a lovely woman. I had met with her a couple of times at a nursing home before she had died. Little by little I began to remember other faces, people who had shared so much of themselves with me and with each other.

"Have you heard from Jerry?" I asked, pleased to remember the name of a man with an impressive beard who'd been a longtime member of the group.

"Not for years," she said. "But you know what? Sometimes it's like I can hear him laughing. It's like I still carry a little bit of them around with me."

I sat with this thought for a moment. Faces flashed in my mind, mostly without names but welcome. Warm feelings flooded in. I wanted more, but I also knew it was important to keep the session focused on her experience.

"Tell me, Debbie, why do you think our group was so meaningful?"

"So many reasons! It felt something like family, I think. Not always loving but important. We really listened to each other. We really learned. And somehow, Irv, you were able to make it safe for us, even when we were sharing difficult things, things maybe we were ashamed or sad about."

"That's lovely. We must have all done a very good job together."

At the end of our hour, Debbie thanked me and handed me a check for four hundred dollars. Taking it in my hand, I froze up. I felt extremely uncomfortable accepting her check.

"Hold on, Debbie," I said. After thinking about it for a few moments, I handed the check back to her and suggested that she pay half of the fee. She gladly tore it up and wrote another.

One day, when Debbie reads this story, I'm sure she will understand why I could not accept the full amount from her. I had done some good work, giving her perspective on her dear friend's death and alleviating her powerful sense of guilt. But she had given me just as much by returning me to that group and that time of my life. I'd had energy and passion, and I'd been remarkably fortunate to land in Northern California at such a fertile moment in the field, when people were suddenly seeking self-knowledge and consciousness raising with such authentic curiosity. There was a sense of openness, of possibility, and we invested ourselves fully in our practices working with patients, in experimenting with new ideas and approaches, and sitting in that sun-dappled, dusty office listening to each other, attuned to one another's challenges and emotions, sharing ourselves.

CHAPTER 18

Judy Steinberg's Birthday

Martha was a thirty-nine-year-old Australian thera-pist who seemed enviably comfortable in her own skin. At the beginning of our session she told me that she had a thriving psychotherapy practice and was close to her mother and her two brothers. After we had spoken for about twenty minutes, I began to grow puzzled. It was nearly halfway through our session, and I still had no idea why she had contacted me. Everything seemed to be going well in Martha's world.

I squinted and listened harder as she told me she had just finished a two-year course of therapy with a psychoanalytically oriented therapist, which she had found useful. I waited for her to turn to problematic areas in her life, but she gave no signs of distress, aside from a brief mention of her parents' divorce and her father's disappearance from her life when she was four years old.

More than once I asked why she had contacted me, but she seemed perfectly content to continue in chitchat for the entire, very expensive hour. I thought I should try even harder to help guide our session someplace deeper, but then she was a professional therapist who certainly knew that patients need to share if they are to get anything out of therapy. The clock continued to run, and my inner questions grew more pressing. What was going on? Why was she so passive? I tried my usual methods to help a patient talk, but each one was strikingly ineffective.

"Martha," I finally ventured, "up to now I've been posing personal questions to you. But we seem to have come to a stalemate. I suggest that you and I switch roles for a bit. Please, I'd like you to pose some questions to me about my life. I promise to answer any question you ask the best I can."

What transpired was silence. I waited. More silence. I gave a bit of a shove. "Ask any question, Martha . . . the deeper, the more personal, the better."

Nothing but silence and her placid gaze. What was her silence saying? Why was this so hard? I began to feel a bit guilty for putting her in such an uncomfortable position. Yet all I saw on her face was tranquility. I continued to prod.

"Your turn to be curious, Martha. Don't be concerned about me. I'm comfortable with any question that comes to mind."

But she gave no response. I'd been using this technique in the hardest cases for several months now, and with nearly every person it had conjured up abundant inquiries. But no matter how I framed it now, Martha remained calm and silent. All my efforts to coax her to speak were unsuccessful and the clock ticked out the hour. I was dumbfounded.

"I'm so sorry, Martha, but our time has run out," I said. "I'm not sure I've been very helpful to you, but I'd very much appreciate your writing to me in the coming days and giving me some feedback about our session." And with that I signed off.

What a fiasco! Not a single question from her. That calm smile never wavered, and my new secret weapon failed miserably. I expected not to hear from Martha again, assuming she would agree that our hour had been a dud.

And yet a few days later her check arrived along with a handwritten note on light blue paper:

Thank you so much for our session, Dr. Yalom. We hit on something very important, I think, a real and deep fear. But it is difficult to grasp. I would be grateful for another session if you would be willing.

I was relieved to hear from her. The riddle of our first meeting had continued to rattle around in my brain. Her words that we had hit upon something very important were surprising, given how unsuccessful I felt the session had been. This amplified the mystery in my brain. Her statement that this pointed to "a real and deep fear" hinted at a much-needed clue. I agreed to meet again and prepared to follow whatever path these clues pointed toward.

Over the months I had agreed to several second sessions, almost all of them when the first session had seemed highly problematic. This certainly felt like one of those cases and, prior to our next session, I read through my notes with heightened energy, hoping to do better.

"I'm glad we're meeting again, Martha," I began when her face appeared. "Today, right now, what are your thoughts and feelings about our last session?"

"I was expecting that question, but it's all so muddy in my mind," she began. "I know I didn't open up. I wanted to but couldn't!"

"Any thoughts as to why not?"

"Maybe I was afraid you'd find out something bad about me. Or maybe I would not be able to open up in the right way."

"I wonder if you, as a therapist, are so used to being the one asking the questions that being in the responder position was a challenge."

That didn't seem to strike a chord for her, so I pushed a little further.

"There was a point at which I asked you to ask me questions. Do you remember that?"

"Yes. That was the worst. I felt so put on the spot, and my mind kind of went blank."

Interesting! I had been thinking that this question served, in part, to relieve some pressure on the patient, to help them let down their guard and allow me to open up a door to some intimacy. With Martha, clearly, it had had the opposite effect. So this role reversal could, in fact, be a frightening challenge. This was a useful revelation. I would have to be more cautious using it in the future. I wanted to ask more about this experience for my own edification but knew it was more important to focus on her.

"Any idea why you had this feeling?"

"Anxiety," she said. "Others have told me that I don't reveal much and just seem calm all the time. But under my skin, trust me, there is no calm. There is raw anxiety. Always has been. I have no real explanation, but my father leaving when I was four years old is central."

"That sounds significant. Can you say more?"

"Maybe there is something ugly about me, something I don't want anyone to see. Maybe that's why my father left. His leaving was a mystery. My mother has always refused to speak about it. And even though I was so young at the time, somehow

I felt that it was my fault. I know that makes no sense, but I can't let go of it."

"What a deep wound, Martha. You were a child, and whatever happened then was *not* your fault."

"But it feels that way. Inside."

"Perhaps he was not prepared to be a father. Most likely we'll never know the truth. But we *can* discover the truth about *right now*. So let's look at us, at you and me. What makes it so difficult for you to speak right now?"

"Fear. There's no other word for it. Fear of you."

"What is there about me that frightens you?"

"Everything. You're famous. Everyone respects you. You can't imagine how frightening you are to me. My professor talked about you all the time, and we used your books in several classes."

Again I hear I am frightening! I've spent so much of my life trying to be gentle and understanding. It surprises me each time I encounter this fear, which has happened far more frequently in the onetime consultations than ever before. I suspect there are a couple of key factors here. Overall I'm meeting with many more people than I have in the past, when I'd see the same patients week after week—so there are many more opportunities to seem scary. There are also many more therapists requesting consultations than in the past, probably because a onetime meeting is affordable in a way that ongoing therapy wouldn't be. And of course therapists are the people most likely to find me intimidating. Add in the pressure of our short time together, and the manifestations of fear and intimidation are compressed: instead of an acclimation period in which a patient gets to know me over a series of weeks, and likely works through whatever fear they might have, they now have to confront it all at once. Whatever the reason, I needed to be cautious and allay these fears quickly.

"I have learned he can be intimidating," I said, "this Dr. Yalom with all his books. How about you call me Irv from now on? Would that help?"

A smile crept slowly across Martha's lips, and she nodded for me to go on.

"I'm hearing you speak of two important and frightening men, your father and me."

She nodded again.

I asked if there were other men in her life, and she let me know that she'd had several relationships, but none had lasted very long. It sounded as if she had difficulty becoming truly close to her romantic partners, maybe to people in general. I asked what got in her way.

"They'll find out what I'm really like," she said. "That I'm just not good enough. That I'm as ugly on the inside as on the outside."

Whoa! Not only was Martha not ugly, she had a warm, welcoming smile and sparkling eyes. I told her so, adding how dreadful it is that women are constantly made to feel inadequate and ashamed of their appearance. This is one of the most consistently psychologically damaging aspects of our culture, and it has only gotten worse over the decades I've been practicing. Society's assessment (by men and women) of a woman's value based on her appearance is deeply ingrained. Looking back over my own writings, I suspect that I have sometimes unintentionally perpetuated this myself, describing female patients' appearance before writing anything else about them. These descriptions are usually positive, but to many readers, these intended compliments may, in an age when we are increasingly aware of power and gender dynamics, come off as placing appearance above substance. I hear echoes of messages Marilyn, in her strongly feminist work, was struggling with through the decades.

Nonetheless, I told Martha she was certainly not ugly.

"Thank you," Martha said. "But I feel . . . what? . . . rotten at the core."

"I suspect you have your father, and maybe others, to thank for that."

"How does one get over it, the shame?" she asked.

I was about to tell her of my own experiences in personal therapy when a slice of memory from long, long ago—something I hadn't thought of in many decades—popped into my mind.

"Martha, the strangest image just came to me. Do you mind if I tell you a story? I'm not sure it will be helpful, but it might be. Worth the risk?"

She nodded.

"Okay, good. Many years ago, when I was about twelve, I lived in a shabby apartment, worse than shabby, over my parents' small grocery store in a very run-down section of Washington, DC. When schools closed for summer vacations, my parents were concerned about all the trouble or danger I might get into, and they spared no expense to send me to good summer camps for two months. One summer I went to Camp Crestmont in Maryland where I had my first girlfriend and, I think, got my first kiss. Her name just floated into my mind—Judy Steinberg. I'm rather stunned that I remember that, actually. I haven't thought of her in decades, but I can picture her perfectly now."

I paused for a moment, wondering at the marvels of the brain, then continued.

"Well, three or four months later I got an invitation in the mail to a party celebrating Judy's thirteenth birthday. Judy lived in Chevy Chase, an upscale suburb outside of Washington, and her parents were apparently very wealthy. My mother drove me to the party and Judy's parents were to drive me home. I recall that after being in Judy's beautiful house I felt crushingly ashamed about living in such a grungy section of town. Later her parents drove me home, with Judy and me sitting in the back seat. Driving into my neighborhood, I began to feel queasy, waves of shame washing over me. My stomach is bothering me now, just remembering this. As we approached my parents' store, my eyes landed on a much nicer home across the street. I pretended that was where I lived and asked them to drop me off there. I walked up the porch steps, praying the neighbors did not open their door and ask what I was doing there. Judy and her parents watched and waited. I turned around and continued to wave goodbye for a few minutes until Judy's parents finally drove off, leaving me standing there, alone with my shame."

Martha and I sat in silence for a couple of moments until I asked, "How do you feel about what I just said?"

"Shocked," Martha said.

"Tell me about your shock," I said.

"I just can't imagine sharing such things about my life with anyone."

"Why not? What do you fear?"

"Not being good enough, I suppose."

"When . . . where . . . did that begin?"

She remained silent.

"Your father left you when you were four. Was that the beginning?"

"That's what my therapist used to say."

"And how did you feel about what your therapist said?"

"It never helped," she said, then lapsed back into silence.

"Let's go back to what just happened in our session. I want to ask again, how did you feel when I described my behavior after my girlfriend's thirteenth birthday party?"

"Gobsmacked. Absolutely gobsmacked."

"By what?"

"By your telling me this story! I've seen videos of your lectures, read your books. Who am *I* for you to share this with? Honestly I'd never dream of sharing that much with a patient. I've just finished two years of therapy, and I don't think my therapist told me that much about herself in those hundred sessions combined."

"Well, she should have! That's a problem with the field, Martha, not with you. I think sharing parts of yourself with your patients is essential to creating a real relationship."

"I'm . . . what? . . . honored, I guess."

"I'm happy to bestow that honor on you! But you're setting yourself so inferior to me. You needn't. We're not so different, Martha, you and I. We're both therapists, dedicated to helping others. And we both had traumatic childhoods that bedevil us."

"But we *are* so different," she replied. "You seem so comfortable just going ahead and telling people about your trauma, your embarrassments. How did you grow beyond the shame?"

"I did it by doing exactly what you are doing today. I decided to get help and saw several excellent therapists. I worked on myself. I am still working on myself."

After a brief silence I said, "Stay with me, Martha. What's happening inside of you?"

"So much. I'm moved, grateful. And I'm full of questions."

"We've still got time for a couple of questions."

"Okay. I feel nosy asking, but what issues are you working on now in your therapy?"

A brief moment of hesitation as I wondered how I could make this information useful to Martha. Actually it seemed quite clear, as the heart of my issues felt so similar in some ways to hers. I plunged in.

"For several months now I've been working on a big challenge. Every day I receive many emails, dozens, whose writers tell me how important my books have been for them, and often what an 'amazing' or 'important' person I am. I realize this sounds ridiculous to complain about, but here's the thing—somehow these emails don't sink in. Like you, perhaps, I cannot fully believe them. No matter how many fill my inbox, no matter how trenchant or glowing they are, they do not penetrate beyond skin deep. I am glad to have helped people with their lives. Very glad. But part of me still feels like that embarrassed boy from a poor family lying about which house he lived in. *If they only knew the real me*, I think, *they would never write.* So really we're working on the same issue. Early life trauma is so hard to extinguish."

"Can I ask one more?"

"Absolutely."

"How did you learn to share so much of yourself as a therapist? Most don't. And as you say, 'it's a problem in the field.' How did you do it?"

I thought about this for a moment. Self-disclosure has been so much a part of my work for decades. But where did that approach come from?

"Two things come to mind, Martha. The first is that when I was training to be a psychiatrist I was in personal therapy with an old-school psychoanalyst who mostly just sat back and listened to me without offering anything of herself. Good old Freudian blank screen, with the occasional nod or 'hmm,' and sometimes a dream interpretation or a bit of free association. She was cold and distant. I lay on her couch four days a week for three years. Can you imagine? Six hundred hours in total. And the only useful thing I learned from her in all those hours was that this was absolutely not the kind of therapist I wanted to be."

"You have succeeded," she said with a laugh, "in not being a blank screen!"

"Phew," I said with a smile. "The second thought is that I was very lucky as a resident to learn from a wonderful psychiatrist, Jerome Frank, at Johns Hopkins. He taught me to lead therapy groups, and one thing he did that was extraordinary was to focus on what was going on between the group members in real time. He would encourage them to share what they felt about things the other members were saying, to be honest, and to speak about their own feelings."

"I know about process groups," Martha said. "We all read your group book in grad school."

"This approach may not seem revolutionary now," I said, "but asking people, therapists or patients, to express what they truly feel about one another was *vastly* different from what most people in the field were doing. Jerry Frank was gentle and inquisitive, and really interested in what the group members were experiencing. I was immediately won over and began leading groups this way. And I guess it evolved over time, becoming my here-and-now focus—first in the groups I led, and then into my approach to individual therapy. Being open about my emotions with patients was the big step. Once I became comfortable revealing my emotional responses, I gradually expanded to include more of myself and my own experiences when it seemed this would be helpful to my patients. It didn't always come easily, sharing my private world. But I worked on it, and often this sharing seems to help build trust between myself and my patients. Now, in these single sessions, I'm trying to accelerate the process. Sometimes it feels quite rushed, but generally if I am open, then my patients are more easily able to be open in return, like in our session today. Maybe this acceleration is part of what made you feel so pressured in our first session?"

"Yes, I think so," said Martha. "My fear of you probably would have come through either way. But I did feel pressured to move faster than I was ready to."

"My apologies for that. Whatever fear you have of me, I want you to remember that we are both just human beings, and both dealing with traumatic childhoods. Your mother may have been marvelous and provided you with a good, stable, and loving home. But how could you not feel the damage your father left behind? So much doubt, so much self-blame. Even that state of unknowing why he left is a real trauma. It's bound to have a strong impact on a little girl."

"Does that mean I'll be struggling like this for the next fifty years?"

"It will improve," I said. "It may never go away completely, but you can work on it starting now. I didn't focus on the impacts of my childhood until much later in life. I had such a powerful bond with my wife, Marilyn, that I was generally grounded in the world and less beset by these fears. Looking back, I have had constant anxiety, which I translated into constant work, with patients, in teaching, and especially in writing. So in a way my marriage and my career protected me, but also prevented me from doing useful exhuming and reprocessing on my childhood trauma. Since Marilyn died I have been faced with it daily, and I am finally addressing it directly in therapy. You have decades ahead of you and can make much more progress than I have, and much sooner."

"How should I begin?"

"I'll send you a couple of referrals to excellent therapists who focus very much on childhood trauma. Try not to shy away from those dark places but explore them bravely. And as you do, please have compassion for that little four-year-old girl you carry inside of you, the one who sits wondering why her father isn't coming home."

CHAPTER 19

Dull Days in London

D ull, dull, dull," were Millie's first words to me. "Everything feels dull. Nothing is working. My marriage is
dull, my courses are dull, my research is dull."

Millie was a thirty-four-year-old Londoner, finishing up
her PhD in clinical psychology. Her face seemed a poignant
canvas, a charming smile layered over with sadness.

"I feel deadened when I wake up every morning," she
continued. "Nothing is working like it should be."

"Tell me more about 'nothing working,'" I asked.

"It's hard to put into words. My husband and I have grown
apart, for one. He's a computer scientist, and totally into his
work. I don't understand his field. And if I'm honest, I don't
care about it. So there's that."

She paused. I nudged.

"And?"

"And I'm bored with my field."

"What about it is boring?"

"Everything. Everything is boring, including myself. Especially myself."

"You've lost interest in becoming a psychologist?"

"Maybe 'having doubts' about it is better. How will I be able to help people if I'm . . ." Her voice trailed off as she struggled for words. Finally she opened her hands as if to say *if I'm like this*.

"I'm sorry this is such a hard time right now," I said. "Can you tell me what you are hoping for in this session?"

"Irv—is it all right if I call you Irv?"

"Of course. I prefer it."

"Irv, I . . ." She went silent for a few moments. "I don't know how to start," she said finally.

"Nothing comes to mind?"

"It's a mess of ideas in my mind. None seem clear right now. Or important."

After another couple of minutes of false starts, each ending in a morass of unknowing grayness, I shifted gears.

"Here's an idea. Why don't you ask me some questions? Maybe my experiences will give us a useful jumping-off point. This way you can help me help you. I'll gladly answer any questions you ask."

She glanced up, a look of surprise on her face.

"*Any* questions? Bold."

"How so?"

"That's a . . . well, I've never heard of a therapist proposing that."

"Let's try it out. What would you like to know about me?"

She thought for a few moments, a small battle playing out on her face between the forces of depression and those of intrigue. Finally the latter won out.

"Somewhere I read that you spent a year in London at the Tavistock Clinic. I'd love to know what that experience was like for you. Maybe it'll help me appreciate my own city more."

"Tricky question, Millie. That was long, long ago, and I have trouble remembering today's breakfast. But let's see . . . I know I chose to go to London that year, late sixties it must have been, because the Tavistock Clinic was one of the most prominent centers for group therapy at the time. I planned to spend my sabbatical year writing a book on group therapy. There wasn't a single decent comprehensive textbook back in those primeval times, and I set out to fix that."

"I know the clinic well," Millie said. "That's one of the reasons I asked. I just finished a year there studying how to run groups. And reading your book, of course. I think we used the fifth edition."

I had been about to encourage her to ask more questions, but her comment stopped me. My experience at the Tavistock Clinic had been similar to my personal psychoanalysis as a resident, a great study in how *not* to do therapy.

"I'm sorry, Millie, did you just say that my textbook was required reading at Tavistock?"

Millie eyed me curiously. "Why wouldn't it be? Isn't it the standard text?"

"It certainly isn't the kind of text I imagined the Tavistock Clinic would ever include in their curriculum."

"Really? Didn't you teach group therapy there?"

I must have started laughing then, because Millie looked even more taken aback.

"I know that sounds like a reasonable question, Millie," I assured her. But I couldn't stop chuckling. This seemed too outrageous to be true, reflecting back on how they had treated me when I was there. Not as an esteemed colleague, nor even as a curiosity. More like a spot of mold encroaching on a nice piece of Cheshire cheese.

"I don't get it. What's the joke?"

"It's just . . . Honestly, they did not have the time of day for me. The culture at the clinic there was so uptight. I doubt they were open to learning anything from anywhere outside the British Empire. Certainly not from an American like me."

"Really? What was it like?"

"Well, they had this very impersonal way of leading groups that was bizarre to me. The group leader would never address any of the individual members. Never. All comments were directed to 'the group,' almost as if there were no actual people in the room."

"And they weren't interested in your research?"

"Not in the slightest. Everything I was uncovering flew in the face of what they were teaching. The more I researched, the more it became clear that it was the connections between the group members that led to the key therapeutic elements I distilled—the installation of hope, altruism, group cohesion—honestly, I can't remember the rest right now."

"Catharsis," Millie offered. "I had a test on this not so long ago, but it's a long list! Interpersonal learning, existential factors, universality . . . a few more."

"Nicely done. I give you a B plus. And a C minus for me, sadly."

"We'll both have to check the study notes later," she said with a smile. "So it wasn't a good year for you at Tavistock?"

"Nope. I had zero colleagueship for the year. Not a single member of the faculty ever reached out to me, shared a meal, or even a decent conversation. It was not much fun, but it was great for working out my ideas and for writing."

Then Millie asked where I'd lived that year, and we got into speaking about the thatched roof home on Redington Road where Marilyn and our three eldest children had lived. I recalled several specific streets and parks in the neighborhood, and Millie helped find the names. I had a sudden memory of the sweet shoppe my son Victor had enjoyed visiting each day after school. What a strange thrill, these long-forgotten bits of my life bubbling up from deep subterranean recesses of memory! There was the sprawling park, Hampstead Heath, down the street, and an ancient cemetery right by our house, where Marilyn and I used to stroll, often stopping to read the barely legible inscriptions on the sixteenth-century tombstones.

"I know that cemetery well!" Millie exclaimed. "I live right around the corner."

"You know, Millie, you're changing in front of my eyes. You're different, you're so much more enlivened than you were just fifteen minutes ago. What gives?"

"It might have something to do with the author of my textbooks chatting away and telling me how archaically uptight the Tavistock Clinic was. Yes, I feel a bit giddy. Can I ask more?"

"Oh yes, Millie. I'm loving this conversation, and not only because you're drawing out sparkling memories I forgot I had but because you seem to be having fun."

"I am."

"Less dull now?"

"Absolutely. Do you have any other London memories?"

"Yes, one more is now poking its way into consciousness. Nothing to do with the psychiatry. It's someone familiar . . . round face, gray hair, a cigar . . . damn, what's his name?

Ah! Alex. Alex Comfort. Haven't thought of him in some years."

"Alex Comfort?" she said with surprise. "You mean the Alex Comfort who wrote *The Joy of Sex*?"

"That's the guy. And the book. Funny, that book sold millions of copies, but Alex always groused about it."

"Why? He must have made a fortune."

"He did. And he gave most of it away. He was interested in everything—what a mind! And he was incredibly prolific, and wrote fifty or so books—novels, poetry, social commentary, literary criticism. But that one got all the attention. That's what annoyed him. Then again, sex sells."

"I remember sneaking that book down off my parents' bookshelf and giggling at all the drawings. I felt so naughty! How did you and he meet?"

"I had a minor role, really. Alex adored my wife, Marilyn, I think because she was both beautiful and a rare person with whom he could discuss both medieval history and contemporary literary theory. Whether it was her looks or her mind, he could not get enough of her, so we saw a lot of him. He was a true genius. And funny. Years later he moved to California, so we saw him there, too. I remember he had blown the fingers off one of his hands somehow, and this fascinated my youngest son, Benjy, who insisted on examining the remaining stubs whenever Alex visited."

Our hour was racing by and, as much fun as I was having revisiting these memories, I needed to refocus on her concerns.

"Millie," I said, "you've certainly got my mind racing. But this session isn't about me. Let's take a few minutes to examine what is going on in the here and now. You came to me with a clear problem, and yet mostly we've been talking about me. Honestly, I'm a little bit worried. Has this been at all helpful for you?"

"Hmmm," she said, taking a moment to think. "Well, as I said earlier, everything has seemed so dull these last few months. I've had no energy. It happens in every setting, and I sensed it seeping in at the beginning of our session. I just couldn't get motivated. But as soon as you started talking about your days in London everything changed, and I felt interested, invigorated even."

"Something shifted."

"Yes, you rejuvenated me somehow."

"Give yourself some credit, Millie. You instigated that change when you asked me about my memories of the Tavistock Clinic."

"True, you asked me to ask you. But not many therapists would have engaged me the way you did. You really trusted me. I guess your opening up made it feel safer for me to . . . what . . . stop thinking about myself so much."

"You took enormous advantage of the opportunity, more than most. Did this challenge feel useful to you?"

"Oh yes. Very much so. At least as far as I can tell right now."

"I'm glad. And it certainly isn't intended as a permanent fix! We haven't had time to talk about your personal therapy, but it would be great if you could work with someone who can help you continue to find joy. I'm going to send you some names after this, okay?"

She nodded, then asked, "May I have one more question, please? It seems risky, offering to answer any question I might have. But you just strolled casually into it. How do you do this?"

"Well, I'm at a point in my life where it's not so difficult. Part of it is no longer caring so much what everyone else thinks about me. I am who I am and at ninety that isn't likely to change a lot. It's also not caring so much what other people in the field think. I have certainly not followed the main directions of psychology or psychiatry—neither short-term symptom-focused work nor psychopharmacological solutions for everything. So I have faced some skepticism and resistance over the years. But I know that I've helped many patients, and that is always the most important thing. I'm revealing more now than ever, and it seems to be working."

"But how did you get there? How did you become able to open up?"

"Honestly, it hasn't been an easy process for me. The ability to be open to others was not built into my personality. Meeting Marilyn, who was so much more extroverted and confident than I am, helped a great deal. And it took a lot of work to lower my defenses, to become honest with myself, and to learn to like myself, flaws and all. Therapy, self-reflection, watching my patients and my children and learning from them all. I wish I had known earlier how important it is, how useful for my patients, for me to be so open. I would have worked harder on developing this capacity when I was younger. But in my training no one ever emphasized that as a skill therapists needed to learn."

"None of my teachers have, either."

"Well, they should. It's distressing that they don't. If there is one thing I've learned from the hundreds of single sessions I've had this last year, it's this: the more I reveal of myself, the more people reveal back to me."

"So why don't they teach it?"

"The powers that be seem to think it is dangerous. Well,

therapists need to be brave! Being truly empathetic requires some emotional risk on our part."

"I hadn't thought of it that way."

"That brings us to a key question. Does becoming a therapist still seem dull? Still having doubts?"

"If I could help others experience this energy, this connection, that would be exciting. It just feels so distant from what we're learning."

"You don't have to do some plodding textbook version of therapy. You have to bring yourself to it, and discover what works for you and what inspires you. If I had to spend a career running groups the way they used to at Tavistock—never connecting, never treating the members as individual human beings—I'd be pretty down, too, and I suspect everything in my life would feel quite dull and cold."

"Dull and cold, yes."

That gave me a thought.

"Millie, I'm writing a book about some of these consultations and we've chosen the title *Hour of the Heart* because of the intimacy and warmth of sessions like this. But the Tavistock approach was more like . . . what's far away from intimacy and warmth? Hour of the . . . what? The foot?"

"Cold foot?"

"That's good. *Hour of the Cold Foot.*"

"Wait . . . *Hour of the Cold Foot in a Soggy Sock.*"

"Excellent!"

"*Hour of the Cold Foot in a Soggy Sock inside a Wet, Muddy, Very Sensible Boot!*"

"The publisher will love it!" I said. "Final question: What did you do with that dull Millie I met a little while ago? The one with a layer of sadness on her face like soot coating some building in a Dickens novel."

"Me? What did *you* do with her?" she said, nearly giggling.

We continued, playfully, for a couple more minutes, but soon our time was up.

"I hate to stop now, but I hope you can take some of this more joyous Millie back into your work and your marriage."

"I hope so, too," she said. "I'm optimistic she'll stick around, with some help. Thank you for reintroducing me to her."

CHAPTER 20

A Terrible Beginning

Sonja, a twenty-six-year-old woman who had just finished graduate school and was beginning her career as a social worker in New Zealand, had had one of the worst starts in life of any patient I've ever encountered. She had emigrated from Bulgaria when she was six years old, with her mother, father, and sixteen-year-old sister. Her parents despised each other so much that they not only slept in different beds but on different stories of their small, crowded, and run-down house in Auckland. Her father slept on the floor in the attic, while Sonja and her mother and sister shared one small bed in a tiny bedroom. Her parents were so consumed with their internecine battle that they gave no emotional support to their children. What attention they offered was abusive, both emotionally and physically, with both parents seemingly using Sonja as a surrogate for pain they wished to inflict on each other. Her older sister, who might possibly have provided some support or buffer for Sonja, fled the family home soon after they arrived in New Zealand and never contacted any of them again.

When there was not active abuse, there was deep and abiding neglect. Sonja was left to fend for herself in extraordinary ways: her parents were uneducated and poor, and Sonja had no one to help her navigate this new country with its strange customs. She was shabbily clothed, constantly hungry, and spoke no English, starting first grade entirely unable to communicate with her teachers or classmates.

Against such long odds, Sonja had grown into an insightful young adult. In exchange for doing some administrative work, the Catholic Church had given her housing in a nunnery, where she had lived throughout her two-year clinical psychology training program. She had maintained some contact with her mother, with whom she hoped to develop a new, better relationship. Her father had died several years earlier. She seemed at peace when we met, eager to engage, and eager to learn as much as possible about her chosen field.

"So many people suffer without anyone to lift them up. I want to be that helping hand," she concluded.

"I am astounded by all you've overcome!" I told her.

"Thank you," she responded with a smile, adding, "Meeting with you feels like a rite of passage."

Imagining her solitude upon immigrating, the lack of parental support, being a stranger in a strange land, I told her a bit of my own isolation as a child, of long hours at the library with piles of books, which were the closest things I had to friends I could bring home.

"Trauma sticks with you," I said. "I'm doing a lot of work on mine now, at ninety. Can you believe it? Fortunately you are aware of it at a . . . just slightly . . . younger age, and it does not have to stop you from doing wonderful things in your life. But you need to remember that it's there and be aware of how it impacts you."

226 • HOUR OF THE HEART

She nodded, seemingly cognizant of all of this.

"Who were you closest to as a child?" I asked, hoping to get more of a sense of her early life.

This stymied her. She searched her mind for a moment but found she could not name a single friend. She had been so pleased when we began speaking, but now her affect changed, saddened.

"Let me rephrase that question," I said. "Who are you closest to in all the world now?"

She looked even sadder and avoided my glance. Slowly she shook her head.

"I had a boyfriend for a while," she said. "And I learned some things about friendship from that. Mostly I learned that I wanted to be treated better."

"And other friends?"

"I don't think I know how," she said.

Oh Sonja! It struck me that she had no close relationships, and perhaps had never had any in her entire life. Even the most self-sufficient people need close relationships. I knew what I had to do. I had to help her understand what it is to share deeply with another person, to know what is possible, so she might become able to create it elsewhere in her life. Therapy often serves as a valuable dress rehearsal for life, with the therapist serving as a rehearsal mate. With this goal in mind, I wanted Sonja to experience intimacy.

"Sonja, let me make an unusual suggestion. Please let's try switching roles for a few minutes. I've been asking you a great many personal questions and now I'd like you to ask me questions about my life and my thoughts. I promise you I'll answer every question you ask. Please give it a try."

Sonja immediately brightened and leaped into the task. "I

heard about your wife's death, Dr. Yalom. Is it all right to talk about your wife? Or is that too hard?"

"No limits on your questions, Sonja. The more personal, the better."

"Can you tell me how you met your wife?"

"I met my wife, Marilyn, when I was fourteen and had just moved from the wretched part of town where I'd grown up to her pleasant neighborhood in Washington, DC. I had been bowling with a classmate—Louie was his name—and when we finished, he said, 'There's a party at Marilyn Koenick's house. Want to go?' I agreed, but when we got there, we saw a mob of teenagers on her porch trying to get through her front door. I was an awkward kid, uncomfortable around crowds, and I was ready to go home, but Louie, who was a bit of a troublemaker, convinced me to climb through the window."

Sonja seemed intrigued. "What did you and she talk about? And what did you do on your first real date?"

I answered her as best I could, telling her about Marilyn's and my shared love of books, and the movies and plays we watched together. Then I encouraged her. "Sonja, I love your asking these questions. You're doing great. What else would you like to know?"

"Dr. Yalom—"

"Irv, please."

"Irv, how did you get interested in psychiatry? And philosophy? You wrote a novel about Nietzsche and one about Schopenhauer and another about Spinoza. What connection did you see between psychiatry and philosophy?"

Quite a shift! What wonderful, bold questions. I answered, wanting to respond with the same degree of sophistication, while also emphasizing interpersonal connection wherever I could.

"Excellent questions. It didn't happen right away. Marilyn and I went to different colleges, hours away from each other. I couldn't stand being so far away, and I rushed through my studies in only three years, taking nothing but the science courses required for medical school so I could establish myself as having a real future in her eyes as quickly as possible. I had to hurry, before she fell for someone else."

"You were scared of this?"

"I was terrified. Well, these classes were mostly rote memorization, with little critical thought and no exposure whatsoever to literature or philosophy." I continued, telling her about entering medical school and choosing psychiatry because it seemed something like literature, and then about encountering Rollo May's book *Existence*, and how that impacted my thinking.

"Thanks to Rollo I saw that many wise people have been interested in big questions around human life and meaning for thousands of years. And I thought there must be a way to incorporate these ideas into our field. But I had no understanding of philosophy at that point. I immediately enrolled in an introduction to philosophy course at Johns Hopkins that met three evenings a week for the entire year. This was one of the most important courses of my entire education. Even now, sixty years later, I can still summon the teacher's face but not his name."

"Thank you! And thank you, Dr. Yalom, for seeing that the troubled mind needs philosophy as much as medicine." Sonja glanced anxiously at her watch and said, "Please, can I still ask another question?"

"Yes, Sonja, but only if I can ask you one last question after that."

She nodded quickly, then launched in, almost voraciously.

"How did you and your wife get to be such great friends? How did you learn to do that? How did the two of you make friends with others? Did you and she like the same people?"

"That one last question has morphed into a lot of good questions, Sonja! It's hard to answer them all, but two thoughts about friendship come to mind. First, Marilyn was the one who made friends for us as a couple, and eventually for our family. Remember, I was the clumsy kid who crawled in through her window, and only after being forced to do it. I still feel that way, a trespasser in finer social circles. She had an ease about her and loved to be out and about, while I was usually a bit anxious and longed to be home reading a book. So I don't know that I have been a great friend maker. But with the close friends I did make over the years, I really cherished them and worked to make those relationships flourish. I called them all regularly, wherever we were in the world, and made sure to visit whenever possible. And I was always open with them, about my hopes and fears—in the way you and I have been today. Friendship takes work, and sometimes risk."

I had meant to end there, my last words sounding a bit like sage advice. But Sonja looked at me so intently, and I felt so connected to her in that moment, that my next thoughts poured out unbidden.

"And now they are all gone," I said. "All of them. And I'm left alone, trying to hold on to memories, while my mind flakes away."

I reached for a tissue and dabbed at my eyes. There was no hiding the emotion that had come over me, and we sat together in silence. Sonja stayed present with me, with dark, gentle eyes.

"And now for my question to you, okay?" I said after a couple of moments.

She nodded, sat up in her chair, and straightened her shoulders.

"My question is: What has our talk been like for you today? What have you . . ."

Before I could finish, tears began to gush from her eyes, and she made no effort to stop them, or her loud sobs. "Oh. Dr. Yalom, thank you, thank you. This is the closest talk I've ever, ever had . . . no one has ever shared so much with me. I'll remember our talk as long as I live. Now I know friendship. Now I know what it's like. Thank you for this feeling."

Sonja let her tears flow and soon my tears began again also, for myself, for my wife and friends gone, and mostly for this young woman, trying so hard to make a whole life after such a terrible beginning.

Several days later Sonja emailed me, grateful for such a transformative meeting. "I only hope, someday, I am able to offer such a powerful experience to some of my clients," she wrote.

"Sonja," I responded, "I am certain that you are going to be a superb therapist. You have this in writing. Whenever you feel doubtful or dismayed, please look at this message from me."

I did not say this lightly. I was deeply moved by all she had overcome and by her passion to learn and to be helpful. And I was impressed by, and grateful for, how she'd stayed present and engaged while I had wept. She deserved support, something she had never received from anyone in her life, and I was happy to give it. Though there are things about myself that I don't like, I do love my desire to help others and I don't hold back from expressing positive feelings toward my patients and students.

My dedication to offering praise and support has a backstory, which I thought about after my correspondence with

Sonja. Many decades ago, soon after my psychiatry training, I applied for a faculty position at Stanford University. I met with David Hamburg, the chairman of the newly formed Department of Psychiatry. After a very brief interview, I was astounded when he offered me, right then and there, the position as an assistant professor. I accepted the next day, after speaking with Marilyn, and went on to spend my entire academic career at Stanford.

I often wondered why he offered me such an excellent position after such a brief interview. I had no track record to speak of, and a tenure-track professorship with significant academic freedom was no small prize. It was thirty years later when I learned the answer. Dr. Hamburg had been packing up his office for our move to a new building and had come upon a letter of recommendation sent decades previously by John Whitehorn, the chair of psychiatry at Johns Hopkins, where I had done my psychiatric residency. Since Dr. Whitehorn had died years before, Dr. Hamburg now felt he was free to share the letter with me. I wasn't sure what to expect. Dr. Whitehorn had been a remarkable teacher, an elder I respected immensely. But he had always been rather distant and had rarely shared a personal word with me during my three-year residency. He was an esteemed professor, admired by us trainees, but also intimidating, ever clothed in a crisp white shirt, brown suit, and tie.

The letter shocked me. The last line read, "Dr. Yalom was an unusually creative student and I consider it likely that he will become a leader of American psychiatry."

I had no idea, none, that he had thought so highly of me. It was a pleasure to finally learn his opinion, but since then I've often thought, "Oh, I wish I had seen this letter years ago." Or better yet, "I wish Dr. Whitehorn had said these words to me personally." It would have radically changed the way I felt about myself, given me greater confidence, reduced my anxiety, made me feel less like an interloper at the university, crawling in through the side window!

And so I made sure to tell Sonja of my enthusiastic feelings for her and her future, a future that will be so much richer than her past. I've learned through the years that we should not be stingy with our praise, not to patients or friends or colleagues. If being privy to people's inner struggles for sixty years has taught me anything, it's that people's outward appearance of confidence and success often has little connection to the way they feel inside. You never know who desperately needs to hear approval or feel love.

CHAPTER 21

A Wonderful Beginning

I ndeed, Sonja had one of the worst starts in life that I've ever encountered. In what struck me as a great coincidence, Richard, with whom I had a consultation the following morning, had one of the best. He was an unusually well-spoken, poised, and handsome forty-eight-year-old Australian man with the look of the middle-aged Paul Newman. I could easily imagine him nonchalantly strolling off a Hollywood set after a day's filming of a movie about Wall Street, his coat slung over one shoulder, his flawless grin catching the golden late afternoon sun.

Self-assuredly taking the initiative in our session, Richard first spoke glowingly of his parents, both of whom had been longtime CEOs of highly successful firms now enjoying the type of retirement one fantasizes about, traveling the world in luxurious style, strolling leisurely through Parisian museums, diving the Great Barrier Reef. He then proceeded to describe how he had followed their example and for the last ten years had been the CEO of a prosperous investment bank.

Richard had lived a happy and unblemished life—valedictorian and class president of a highly regarded college, then an outstanding business school student. Moreover, he had been happily married for twenty-five years to his childhood sweetheart, who had graduated cum laude from an outstanding women's college. Together they had three beautiful children.

Despite that amazing grin and the enviable life story, Richard was contacting me for help. Presumably this man who appeared to have everything felt lacking for something. Though he responded fully and eloquently to my every inquiry, twenty minutes into our session I still felt entirely in the dark about why he had sought my help. Perhaps because he seemed so unperturbed, I, too, relaxed and patiently waited for his mask to crack and for a more distressed expression to emerge. His smile and confidence lulled me into a sense of ease such that I did not push to use our time as effectively as possible right away. I did not dig quickly, asking what was troubling him. Was it deep self-doubts? The impossible challenge of measuring up to his parents? Unfulfilled daydreams of playing in the finals of the Australian Open? Or did he harbor some kind of shame? Was he mesmerized by fetish pornography, struggling with tabooed temptations? Stranger things have been revealed to me in this room.

"So far, Richard," I finally ventured, "your situation in life seems wonderful. You've accomplished so much, and your parents must be purring with pride."

"Oh yes! Purring. Purring loudly."

"But, still, you've contacted me, a psychotherapist on the other side of the world?"

Richard grinned that disarming Paul Newman grin but said nothing.

"Because . . . ?" I nudged.

"Because," he responded at length, "there are tempestuous questions swirling in my mind—questions that belong in everyone's mind, buzzing for attention."

"Say more," I encouraged, intrigued.

"I'm referring to the questions that really matter. Questions that I've ignored or pushed away my whole life until recently. Questions that everyone ignores. Penetrating questions."

"Questions such as . . . ?"

"Such as 'Why is there something rather than nothing?'"

"What?" I asked in an almost squeaky voice.

"Why, instead of boldly facing big questions, have I lived the life of a tin soldier, awaiting the bell of the stock market announcing the daily race for golden coins? There are the other vital questions, too." Before I could inquire, Richard continued. "What was there before the Big Bang? How can matter arise from nothing? And what is infinity?"

Richard's questions caught me completely off guard, and for a moment I was speechless. I reached to the realm of philosophy for a response, but nothing came quickly to mind. Richard paid my silence no heed and plowed forward. "Be it understood, Dr. Yalom, that I plead guilty. Guilty of desertion. Guilty of ignoring such vital questions. Instead, what I have done with my life is to bow shamefully to the hourly clangs of the stock market. Money, money, money. More and more I loathe myself for my greed, for grasping for gold."

"Let's explore that for a moment," I said, recovering my inner balance. "Surely your successes have done some good. I suspect you've helped many others fare better, buy houses, raise families."

"And in so doing I have helped distract them from these important questions," he responded, still smiling.

"Okay," I said. "But on some level, mustn't most people fight for dollars in some way? I fully embrace these big questions, but why beat yourself up for putting food on the table?"

"But *I* didn't need to fight. With all of the resources and privilege I was born into, why couldn't I do better?"

I imagined him lining up every morning with his troop of fellow "tin soldiers" in thousand-dollar suits and Italian calf-skin shoes, awaiting the bell to announce the battle for filthy lucre, and I began to feel sad for him. Without doubt he needed help and I slid back into my familiar role as helper. I had often thought about and written about existential issues, and I should be an excellent therapist for someone with Richard's philosophical quandaries. And yet, as I sought my tools, I could not find them. Most of my philosophical inquiries have focused on ideas of how to live meaningful lives, how to apply the thoughts of great thinkers to our daily existence. Richard's questions were so abstract, so intangible—what was before the Big Bang? These seemed more in the province of physicists or theologians. For a moment I was bereft of ideas. Then I pulled my focus back into the space between us. My task was not to answer these questions but to help Richard understand why they were so important to him, why he was avoiding them, as he put it, and how he might face them.

I began with a modest suggestion. "You know, Richard, these pursuits aren't necessarily mutually exclusive. Why should one rule out the other?"

"I don't understand. Can you spell that out?"

"What prevents you from doing both? I mean, why not explore these vivid metaphysical questions *and* continue the daily work that enables you to support your family?"

"Say more."

"Let's examine some options. You certainly aren't the first

to grapple with these mighty issues, so you could begin by reading deeply. For guidance you might enroll in evening philosophy courses at the University of Melbourne or perhaps form a small discussion group of like-minded others. I doubt you'd have trouble engaging a local underpaid philosopher to lead the group."

"Intriguing," he said. "But very small, I think."

"Okay. Let's step it up a bit. Why not fund an Australian think tank to discuss and research these great questions? You have the financial resources. Imagine the intellectual resources available, the many great minds in your country and elsewhere who would want nothing more than to give up teaching and devote themselves to pure metaphysical exploration."

This caught his attention, and so for the remainder of our session he and I imagined the birth of such a metaphysical think tank. We talked of the impact such a center could have, how the research might happen, and how the new ideas might be disseminated to others throughout society—lecture series, podcasts, and newsletters on the meaning of life sent to everyone from CEOs to bank tellers. It was heady stuff, and I was more energized at the end of the hour than I had been in months.

The high of that exciting brainstorming lasted several hours. Then, later that night, it came crashing down. I became aghast at my work with Richard. Was the dream of founding a think tank all that psychotherapy could offer a patient in need? Is my field so bankrupt? What Richard needed were actual insights, applicable to his life, not a legacy project in which to invest his money. Perhaps I had been caught up in fantasizing of what having such enormous resources would allow me to do. But that was not, I was now certain, what Richard the patient had needed. I soon felt full of shame. A windstorm of thoughts swirled through my mind. Why hadn't I confronted Richard with his lack of gratitude for what his parents had provided him? And why had I not responded to Richard's dismissive remark about the daily greedy race for gold coins? After all, those were the coins that had provided him and his children the best possible education on the planet, coins that provided him an understanding of the very meaning of the word *metaphysics*. Abraham Maslow, I thought, might be having a good laugh at me right now.

Or perhaps I could have offered Richard different perspectives that would help shape his thinking. What value was there in addressing these questions if they don't result in real change? How, for instance, would the answers to his metaphysical questions offer his children better lives? How might he prevent them from using their privilege to repeat the same experience he has had? And what about kindness and mercy, equality, opportunity, and justice?

The next day, as I continued to ponder what I could have and should have said to Richard, the face of Dagfinn Føllesdal glided into my mind. Dagfinn, a philosophy professor at Stanford and in Norway, his home, had been my good friend for many years. I had loved sitting in on his Stanford courses on Husserl and Heidegger, important twentieth-century philosophers. He is a divine lecturer and has the clearest and keenest mind I had ever encountered. Dagfinn's wife, Vera, had died only a few months after Marilyn died, and Dagfinn had been planning to visit and stay with me for a few weeks so that we could deal with our grief together. I had very much been looking forward to hosting him and having deep conversations that might be healing to both of us. But COVID had forced him to postpone his trip.

Suddenly, a brainstorm—perhaps Dagfinn might help! There was no limit to Dagfinn's creativity. I emailed him immediately, hoping he might offer me suggestions for thinking further about the connections between philosophy and psychiatry, and specifically how to help Richard engage in such metaphysical thought, and square that with the other exigencies of his life. Having sent this message, I embarked on my daily walk to Marilyn's bench.

Almost every day, around 5:00 p.m., as I push my walker down the park's packed-earth path, a man in a purple sweater rides past me on a bicycle and nods in a friendly fashion. There is something very familiar about this man. Every time he passes me, he nods, and I always nod back, pretending that I know him. But who is he? I cannot place him in my fading memory. On this particular day, however, much to my surprise and very much unlike me (for deep down I am very shy), I did something quite different. As he bicycled past me I called out loudly, "Stop! Please stop. I want to ask you something."

He stopped his bicycle, dismounted, and, with a big, warm smile on his face, walked it back to me.

"Hello," I greeted him. "We pass each other on this path so often and I know that I know you. Forgive me, but now at the age of ninety, I'm having some memory problems. Can you tell me your name? I'm Irv Yalom."

"Oh Irv, I know you well," the bicyclist said. "I'm Marvin, and you were my teacher. Not too many years ago, I attended a course on philosophy and psychiatry that you gave with Dagfinn Føllesdal at your home. You were a big influence on me, an influence in many ways. I've since gotten my PhD, and I now teach philosophy at Stanford. Also, I liked your home and this particular neighborhood so much that I bought a house two blocks away."

"And you bike here often?"

"Never miss a day—I take an hour's ride just before dinner."

We spoke for several more minutes, and he told me how much he enjoyed the courses he was teaching, particularly to undergraduates.

"I'm so glad to be reacquainted, Marvin. Fair warning, though—I may not remember your name next time you pass by."

"I'll be sure to remind you," he said with a smile.

What an extraordinary encounter. I have passed this man and nodded to him in silence countless times, perhaps two or three times each week for several years, and I've always been perplexed by who he is. And today, immediately after writing a letter to Dagfinn, I suddenly and very uncharacteristically called out to him and asked his name, only to learn that he was a student in the class that Dagfinn and I taught together decades before. Surely this was more than coincidence.

The idea of implicit memory resurfaced, and I chose to lean in and see what was there. Perhaps thinking about Dagfinn earlier had primed me to focus on Marvin as he rode by on his bike. Some part of my mind had been aware that there was a connection between us, even if I could not remember it explicitly, and I called out to him without conscious choice. Marvin had then reminded me that Dagfinn and I had taught a whole course on the intersections of philosophy and psychiatry, precisely where I was stuck with my patient Richard. Ah, the mind. What a marvel, even in decline.

I woke the next morning to a message from Norway. Dagfinn had been out walking to visit his wife Vera's grave. Two old men, then, ten thousand miles apart, missing their mates. He made some observations about our mutual circumstances and bemoaned the impossibility of coming to visit. Regarding

Richard, he suggested that I not attempt to "fix" anything directly with philosophical suggestion. Rather, he noted, Richard would need to find his own way toward such study, ideally through a particular area of his life that moved or puzzled him. For Dagfinn it had been the prospect of marrying Vera. Prior to that Dagfinn had been a mathematician, but when faced with marriage he had begun to read ideas about marriage in various religious traditions, which had led to a lifetime of philosophic inquiry.

He was right, I thought, that I could not simply propose directions of thought for Richard. Moreover, Richard could not simply appoint others to do the research, assign managers to the project, as he would at work. No think tank then—Richard would have to discover these things for himself. Perhaps I could help pique his curiosity and give a gentle push in one direction or another. During the next few days, I thought about a great many things I might have—should have—discussed with Richard were my old brain more nimble. Why were these great questions of such concern to him? Do they shape the way he relates to his wife? Are they born of concerns for his grandchildren? His unborn great-grandchildren? Would answers to such metaphysical questions help him make this world a better place? What kind of world does he want for his descendants? How might he absorb the wisdom and loving contributions of Christ, the Buddha, the Dalai Lama?

Oh, I so much hoped he would ask me for another session. Now I felt fully equipped! I had abundant responses to Richard's search among the great metaphysical questions. What a relief! Yes, yes, psychotherapy has some answers after all—the kind of personal existential thoughts that make Richard and, indeed, all of us truly rich in spirit!

Alas, my satisfaction and certainty were short-lived. A

powerful inspiration early in my career, as I'd told Sonja, was that great minds had been working on these grand questions about life and meaning for thousands of years and that their observations might be of assistance to people in despair. On the one hand there was undoubted value in bringing these ideas to psychotherapy, as so much of this wisdom was helpful to those in distress. On the other hand, perhaps people have been working on these questions for thousands of years precisely because no one has been able to provide sufficient answers. Perhaps such insoluble questions are eternal. Perhaps agonizing about them is our fate, an inescapable aspect of the human condition.

Alas, my mind continues to slip, my awareness perhaps shifting more to the implicitly remembered, away from explicit crisp reasoning. Maybe I will unintentionally stumble on some answers for myself, but I will have to leave it to future generations of therapists and philosophers to grapple further with how psychotherapy best navigates these big questions.

CHAPTER 22

Dementia, Ah Dementia

As I spoke to Jonathan, a primary care physician in Southern California, I was fixated on his every word. His challenges mirrored my own so closely. Jonathan told me his memory was growing more tattered day by day and week by week. The decline had become noticeable about a year before, first as he struggled with people's names and then as his daughter noticed he was repeating himself often in conversation. This had sped up during the previous four months and had gotten to the point that both of his adult children had recently suggested it was time for him to consider retiring. Hearing this had been a shock. Jonathan still felt able to practice medicine competently, but he knew the writing was on the wall.

Hard thoughts plagued him constantly. Was this normal old age mental decline? Or a more aggressive Alzheimer's type dementia? How quickly would his mind decay? Who would he be if he were not working? How would he pass the time? His wife had passed away some time ago, and his children were off living their lives elsewhere. He had friends but was too ashamed to reveal his decline and had been avoiding them. What could he do? And why continue living, only to have senility take away his memories, his work, his friendships—all the things he loved? Suicide, he told me, seemed far preferable to a slow hobble into death.

I could not offer any easy solutions, of course, but I empathized deeply with Jonathan and shared my own fears. Together we looked at some changes that he might make, such as trying to let go of his shame so that he might share his experience with his loved ones. They were far more likely, after all, to offer support and empathy than criticism. We also looked directly at the issue of suicide, about which Jonathan had thought seriously. He assured me that he had no intention of ending his life in the near future but wanted my thoughts. I told him that I did not find the idea of ending one's life anathema, particularly if one were facing a terminal condition. I believe I mentioned Nietzsche's critical idea that one should "die at the right time," and possibly, I don't remember for sure, mentioned that Marilyn had ultimately chosen to end her life with the assistance of a physician once the pain became insufferable. It was a powerful conversation for both of us, I believe, and I found myself jotting many notes on my pad. Toward the end of the session I also found myself thinking, *What help can I offer him when I cannot help myself?*

I ended the session feeling very discouraged for Jonathan. Perhaps if we'd had more time together, were I younger and able to commit to ongoing therapy, I could have offered real assistance. Part of me felt this way. But another voice countered this, assuring me that even if we had more time, I might provide company on the journey of memory loss but little else. We might reflect on lives well lived, on family, on career success. But this might be cold comfort in the face of our decline, as we both sauntered toward the grave.

And in this single hour? All I could ultimately offer was a moment of connection and the names of several excellent therapists. Nothing more.

Every day some incident occurs that reminds me of my own future, my own descent into dementia, my own despair. And perhaps my own suicide. *Suicide*. While the thought of ending my life does visit me occasionally, I rarely use that stark word in my personal musings. I use more acceptable terms, like . . . like . . . how annoying! My aging brain has blocked me from coming up with a more palatable word. I abandon the search and return to the question of my own future as a therapist.

I cannot imagine my life without helping others. What am I if not a therapist? And what if I am not a teacher and writer, for these must someday end, too. Well, I'm a father of four children, a grandfather of eight, and now even a great-grandfather, twice over. And as I mentioned, not a day passes without emails from grateful readers telling me how important my writing has been to them. I wish I could find more comfort in this than I do. This has become a frequent topic in my personal weekly therapy, and I feel great empathy for my therapist as she struggles to comfort me. So I am many things to many people. But my own experience of each day has become much diminished.

Clearly my session with Jonathan stirred up deep thoughts. When he and I finished, I reached for my handwritten notes of key points of the session and prepared to dictate a summary, as I always do. But I was distracted by three phone messages, all of which seemed to urgently need my immediate attention. Twenty minutes later I turned back to my session with Jonathan. I glanced at my notes, waiting for them to jump-start my memory, as they inevitably do. But not this time. I could not recall anything of my session with Jonathan. Not a single detail of the hour-long conversation we had just had. I knew we had talked. I remembered preparing for the session, walking down the path from the house, even sprinkling some water on the bonsai trees by my office entrance. And then, nothing. Not a single image until the phone calls I'd responded to after the session. My notes indicated we had had a thorough and important discussion. But I simply could not recall *any* of it.

I was frozen with wonder and alarm at my empty mind. I looked again at my notes, but they were useless. My handwriting was as disgraceful as usual and no matter how hard I peered, the words were a total mystery. What *had* we discussed during our intensive hour-long consultation? I was absolutely certain that we had had a compelling discussion. Moreover, I could make out the phrase "possible teaching story," which meant it had been fascinating in some way, and it was all the more important that I recapture our hour.

But I could recall nothing. This had never happened to me before. My first thought was to chalk it up to further forgetfulness, but that is not the way my memory impairment has manifested itself thus far. I have forgotten details, such as many people's names and faces, appointments with friends and patients, as well as thousands of stories from my life and those that others have shared with me. But I have never had a recent chunk of time just disappear. As I searched my mind for the next half hour, I experienced a whirlwind of emotions: alarm, irritation, fear for my future.

I was astonished at my seemingly complete amnesia. Where did all that information, that *experience*, vanish to? The feeling was surreal, as if some science fiction novel were playing out in my brain, or *on* my brain, and I was simultaneously observer and subject. How deeply strange—unsettling but also somehow enticing.

Only later, looking back upon those thirty minutes, could I make some sense of these unmoored sensations and of what had perhaps happened. I began to frame it as *one part of me* choosing to blot out my memory of the session in order to protect myself. Jonathan's situation reflected back my own uncomfortably. His thoughts about whether he needed to quit his work, about his identity, and his shame in admitting his decline, all these struck close to home for me. Too close. So in forgetting, I mused, I was effectively preventing myself from facing the threatening details of our consultation. Or perhaps more accurately, *one part of my mind was hiding something from the rest of me*. Yes, that seemed a better way to put it. But as soon as I framed the issue in those terms, an annoying question arose: *Whose mind is this, anyway?* That thought was particularly dizzying, and I sensed an inner voice whispering softly, *Stay away from that question!* But I could not stay away; rather I tried to sit with the idea that part of me is protecting me from myself. *It's for your own good*, I imagined one me saying to another me.

What a strange mind we have. Or should I say, what a clever mind? A mind that had somehow partitioned itself, such that one part had chosen to forget something that the other part knew. Fantastic! There was a battle going on just at the edge of consciousness. But what part of the mind was conscious? First one part and then the other, perhaps. I continued examining this phenomenon, but it was a slippery process. One part would explode into awareness for a moment or two and then be immediately obscured by another part, who saw it as its job to keep the first part from being noticed. Add to this the fact that the only tool I had with which to investigate was the very mind I was attempting to examine. How could I trust what I observed? Even now I grow dizzy as I try to explain this to myself. As I write these last sentences *another* part of my mind shouts, *This is too complex. It's not worth it. Think about something else! Write about something else!*

I stepped back and then tried to sneak up on it, seeking a softer, less directed approach. What had I been thinking or doing before the missing session? Might there be hints among the memories of breakfast, of walking down the path, of watering the bonsais? Neuroscientists would say my memory of the session was not lost but *hidden*. But hidden by whom? From whom? Feeling a bit as if I were drowning, I sought help. I called a close friend, David Spiegel, a psychiatric neurobiological scientist, hoping he could shed some light on this and tell me if it were even possible to have a mind partition itself in this way.

"Sure, Irv," David said, "our brain is complex. There are different parts at play. Recall your neuroanatomy. First think the limbic system that manages emotion and memory. It can hide information and flood you with feelings. It can also inhibit the formation of memories and impact attention. In Freudian terms, which serve as a pretty good analogy, this is the *id*.

"And then, think *ego*, the posterior cingulate cortex and the medial prefrontal cortex, parts of the default mode network. These manage self-reflection and selfhood.

"Finally, think of the prefrontal cortex, which conducts tasks, makes plans, thinks, writes, understands, looks after others. Think *superego*. French analysts call it *surmoi*, the part that is over me. So even in the terminology there are distinct parts, a 'you' and a part of you that is 'over you.'"

David's explanation helped, both the specific information and having someone familiar and trusted to speak with. It was calming to know that the brain does in fact have the potential to bring different areas to focus and to hold multiple intentions simultaneously. And yet knowing that a neurological explanation is possible was not entirely satisfying. This all began when I obliterated my recall of an hour-long consultation I had just concluded. Who was this "I" concealing something from "me"? Were there two entities inside of me? No, obviously there were more than two. There is a third, the "I" who was writing this sentence and was influenced by the existence of the other two.

Only later, over the next few hours, did the full details of my meeting with Jonathan seep back into my consciousness. It was as though I had a caring, overseeing parent in my mind who, as I was about to dictate my summary of my consultation with Jonathan, decided that some of this material would be too painful for me and pieced out little by little what I was allowed to remember. That caring parent part of my mind then entered into an epic struggle with an adult part of my mind, which was set on the task of caring for my consultee, Jonathan, focusing on his story and making sure to send him references. I could feel the struggle, rumbling powerfully inside. Should I take care of myself by forgetting or take care of another by remembering?

And now, should I take care of the self who doesn't want to think more about my crumbling memory? Or should I attend to the self who wishes to write about my experience, so this strange territory might be less frightening for others when they reach it themselves? Or the many other selves, fragmented, floating in my brain and body?

Another self, powerful and benevolent, now emerges upon the scene. It is a self who wishes to protect you, the reader, from drowning in the mayhem of me, the writer. I fight to hold it at bay, because I long to share with you. I spend my days imagining what thoughts to offer. In many ways I make sense of my living through writing, which does not solve, but has often seemed to lessen, the isolation of existence. But now I know I must save you from the confusion swallowing me. Hence these two last gentle words:

THE END

Afterword

by Benjamin Yalom

My father stopped seeing patients soon after the unsettling session with Jonathan. So this is indeed *the end* of his work with patients. But it is not the end of his writing. He is now deep in the middle of what he claims will be his final book. Given his struggles with memory and difficulty sustaining focus for hours on end, as he used to, this is probably true. But if you'll join me here behind the scenes, you'll notice a bit of amused eye-rolling among friends and family members, because he has been adamantly stating that *"this* is the last one" for at least fifteen years, and yet the ideas, and the books, have kept on coming.

Many of the stories in this book, *Hour of the Heart*, examine how powerful it can be to center therapy in the relationship between therapist and patient, and the ways that a therapist's openness can be transformative in therapy, from the here-and-now approach to the revealing of stories from the therapist's life. Time and time again this personal sharing helps these patients discover intimacy and grow in important ways. In my own nascent practice, I have found this sharing to be very powerful. And yet, my father often laments, the field writ large does not embrace these techniques.

I am entering the field just as my father departs, and I, too, am struck by the same strange disconnection. I hear often from students that reading *Love's Executioner* or *The Gift of Therapy* was the reason they decided to become a therapist, or that these books gave them permission to believe they *could* become a therapist. Through these and other books, my father's exploration of the therapy process has been extremely influential. Still, few training programs emphasize his type of interpersonal here-and-now work. The therapist's self-disclosure, particularly when revealing any personal information, is viewed with suspicion, to be avoided most of the time. This is confusing for many students, who begin their training inspired to work on a deeply personal level with patients, only to be cautioned against that kind of intimacy.

Where does this challenge lie? One would think that, evidenced by a great deal of success, these techniques would be taught pervasively. I suggest that there are many impulses that fight against the idea of therapists opening themselves up so fully in session with their patients. Without going into comprehensive detail, here is a brief, certainly incomplete list of some of the most powerful ideas that argue against such disclosure:

- The historical medical model of psychiatry, in which psychiatrists had to be seen as experts,
- The lingering power of Freud's blank-screen approach,
- Fear that if therapists open up too much, their patients will ask them uncomfortable or embarrassing personal questions or in other ways pry into their privacy,
- Fear that romantic or other inappropriate feelings may arise between patient and therapist (note that this may be exacerbated by gender relationships, and may feel particularly perilous for female therapists),

- Fear that if therapists allow themselves to open up, they may be overwhelmed by countertransference, distorting their objective view of their patients,
- The prevalence of short-term "evidence-based" and manualized therapies with clearly delineated steps, which largely view therapists as interchangeable,
- The idea that any focus on the therapist rather than the patient must inevitably be self-indulgent and not in the patient's best interests,
- And finally, as relates to my father specifically, a sense that he must be a bit of a magician and that these techniques work for him in ways they wouldn't for others. (Don't believe it! The essential exhortation is simply for us to be open, honest, and human with our patients.)

These ideas explain some of the resistance to therapist self-disclosure. But I also think that the truth, as it comes to the training of therapists, is a little more complex and a little more hopeful. While few therapy programs specifically teach a here-and-now model, aspects of it—especially examining what is happening in real time between the therapist and patient, as well, possibly, as their partners and/or family members—*have been incorporated into other popular therapeutic approaches*, from psychodynamic to mindfulness-oriented therapies, attachment-based approaches, and couple and family modalities. In several of these there is space for the therapists to open up and give honest emotional feedback, reflecting how they feel about what is happening in therapy sessions and asking how it feels for the clients to experience being seen deeply by the therapist. This type of emotional disclosure has many labels, with variations of terms such as *metaprocessing, congru-ence*, and *authenticity*. For the most part, these models do not work *primarily* with the relationship between therapist and pa-tient, but the key elements of openness and honest exchange are disseminating through the field.

It's the relationship that heals. My father alludes to this "mantra" often. As it turns out, this is no simple personal philosophy, and decades of research now back up this core idea quite powerfully. There are hundreds of theories and approaches to psychotherapy, and knowing what *kind* of therapy you want to seek or practice can be overwhelming. But dig a little deeper into the data about what leads to successful therapy outcomes and the results are pretty startling: the biggest factor in success is the patient's degree of motivation. Depending on the study, this motivation accounts for 40 to 50 percent of the outcomes and is essentially outside the therapist's control. Among the things therapists can impact, *by far the most important is the therapeutic alliance, the relationship between the therapist and patient.* This accounts for 30 to 50 percent of therapy's success or failure. Beyond these two, the particular type of therapy and the particular therapist's skill split up the scant remaining 10 to 20 percent.[*] Given all of this, it seems clear that learning to build the relationship as part of the technique is highly compelling. And that is exactly what

---

[*]   While there is some variance, these numbers represent the trend. For more on the meta-analysis, see C. Flückiger, A. C. Del Re, B. E. Wampold, and A.O. Horvath, "The Alliance in Adult Psychotherapy: a Meta-Analytic Synthesis," *Psychotherapy* 55, no. 4 (2018), 316–40; also Allison L. Baier, Alexander C. Kline, and Norah C. Feeny, "Ther-apeutic Alliance as a Mediator of Change: A Systematic Review and Evaluation of Research," *Clinical Psychology Review* 82 (2020).

my father is doing with all of these self-revelations: in revealing tender parts of himself, he offers a model of how to be open and vulnerable, as well as an invitation for his patients to reciprocate.

And yet most approaches to psychotherapy focus very little on the building of this relationship, treating it as something that is either *there* or *not there*. Given the abundant evidence that indicates that the alliance between therapist and patient is by far the most important factor in successful therapy, this seems deeply self-defeating.

My father's approach to building connection is not the only way to create this bond. For instance, patient and therapist may bond over the joint project of helping the patient. Or the therapist's intense and unflagging interest may in itself feel inviting and powerful enough. Or one may be drawn to the therapist simply by their generally warm and empathetic presence, something along the lines of a surrogate parent, a stronger, wiser other. Each of these is embedded in one or more theories. But the most natural, familiar, and seemingly effective of these, being deeply connected in intimate relationship together as in the stories of this book, remains viewed with deep suspicion.

Why do we hobble ourselves, avoiding this most human, and most familiar, of relationships? Because it is too difficult? Too perilous? Because it requires too much emotional resilience on the part of the therapist? These seem to me poor answers. We must instead be brave enough to become *acrobats of the heart*,* willing to engage intimately, and share deeply, with our

---

* A nod to the theater maker Stephen Wangh's brilliant book with this title, which studies physical approaches actors can use to navigate embodying the difficult and fluctuating emotional terrain of their characters.

patients. My experience has been that some therapists do just this—we let our patients matter to us, and we share of ourselves—yet we often do so cautiously, feeling as if we were breaking some taboo rather than embracing this powerful approach.

"What is it like to have a psychiatrist as a father?" I have been asked this countless times. The people asking have had all sorts of preconceptions and perspectives: there have been those skeptical of psychotherapy (as if I were raised by a con man), those concerned that I was under a mental-health microscope throughout my childhood (and must have suffered as a result), and those who perhaps assumed I had been taught secret powers of psychological manipulation (and viewed me as something of an oddity best kept at a distance). In general, I've responded that I can't give a very insightful answer as I've never had another, non-psychiatrist father with whom to compare. This is just the world I know. And yet it has not been without its challenges. When I was a teenager, a major newspaper ran a large photograph of my father, under the bold headline THE UMPIRE OF REALITY. Imagine having that official statement hang over you, particularly as a cocky adolescent, certain that you know more than everyone else and that your old-fashioned parents are hopelessly out of touch.

As my father mentioned earlier, I indeed avoided the field of psychology for decades in large part because I did not want my professional life to be one of fighting for light under his very long shadow. I was drawn instead to theater and founded foolsFURY, a vibrant and irreverent experimental performance ensemble based in San Francisco. For twenty years we made beautiful and outrageous art, taught workshops for young and old, produced festivals to support other artistic voices, toured, and generally exploded the idea of what theater could be in the twenty-first century. It was a remarkable experience. It also proved, as I got older, to be incompatible with being the father of three small children. Nonetheless, it quite literally took the shutting down of all the world's stages (thank you, COVID) for me to seriously consider changing careers. Then, with time to reflect, I realized that the most important part of the theater was the sense that through all of the rigorous rehearsals, long hours, occasional performances, and deep personal searching, we were growing as people and helping others to do the same. That was what really mattered. Seen in this light, what it means to have a psychiatrist as a father is that embedded deep within me is the drive to help others become richer, fuller human beings. The best tools I know for this are theater and psychotherapy.

I write all of this not to center my own story but in an attempt to share my experience of my father with all of you as best I can, and to honor the part of this book that is about his personal journey as much as it is about therapy. His insistence on intimate reflection is an inheritance I take to heart, and finishing this book, I want to share some last tender images. Let's watch him together now, shall we? He has finished his sixty years of seeing therapy patients, and his memory has flaked away, leaving only a tattered scaffolding. And yet he continues onward, stooped, gray-bearded, the expression on his face a combination of gentle and anxious and always and ever curious. Panama hat on his head, he pushes his walker slowly a bit farther down the path, glancing from side to side, observing, seeking out things to share with us.

His work has been being in caring, intimate relationship with patients, and together using that closeness to examine the big issues of what it means to be human. He has written eloquently about his approach in many books, but the specific mechanisms are less important than the goals. Ultimately his is a therapy of human connection, of letting others matter to us deeply, of seeking meaning and sharing ourselves in the richest and most useful ways possible. Let us take this legacy and strive to encounter one another truly—therapists, patients, fellow humans—in all of our rich, flawed complexity.

Acknowledgments

Irvin D. Yalom acknowledgments:

Many people were critical to the writing of this book, starting with my agent, Sandra Dijkstra; editor, David Groff; and my assistant–guardian angel, Joseph Monzel. Both Eve Yalom and Tracy LaRue Yalom read several early chapters and offered thoughtful feedback, as did many others, all of whom must forgive me for my failing memory. Lastly, I offer an enormous debt of gratitude to my many patients, those who inspired these pages and the hundreds of others over the decades who have filled my work and life with meaning, insight, and endless fascination.

Benjamin Yalom acknowledgments:

I am deeply indebted to many people for helping me grow into who I am today, with a variety of skills and experiences that went into coauthoring this book. First, deep gratitude to those who taught me to write, beginning with my mother, Marilyn Yalom, whose passion for knowledge—always expressed with excellent grammar—resonates through these pages. Thanks also to those at the Iowa Writers' Workshop who helped me hone my voice and skills, particularly James McPherson, Marilynne Robinson, and Frank Conroy, as well as Connie Brothers, without whose encouragement I would never have gotten over my imposter complex enough to attend. Gratitude also to Doug Dorst, collaborator and friend, who has influenced me more than he knows.

Thanks to all the amazing artists and board members I worked with during twenty years of foolsFURY Theater company for helping me better understand the complexities of human nature, desire, creativity, and emotion. Gratitude to those other theater makers who took me under their wings, and helped me to think better and dream bigger, especially Paul Walsh, Corey Fischer, Naomi Newman, Terry Griess, Mary Overlie, and Anne Bogart.

Deep appreciation to those teaching me to be a therapist, especially Thomas Stone Carlson (who keeps exhorting that we therapists *can do better!*), Allison Brownlee (the most encouraging and supportive supervisor I could ask for), and Scott Wooley. Victor Yalom and Tracy LaRue Yalom have offered constant support and perspectives on working with my father's techniques. And Shelly Nathans and Jane Mathisen have spent years with me working on my own brain.

This book would never have seen the light of day without our brilliant agent, Sandra Dijkstra, and her remarkable team, Elise Capron, Andrea Cavallaro, Nick Van Orden, and Jennifer Kim. Deep thanks also to Sarah Haugen and Ezra Kupor at HarperCollins for shepherding us through the process. Additional critical editing, feedback, and research came from David Groff, Angela Santillo, and Joseph Monzel.

Finally, my love to the family, who put up with me through the last two years, and who will be stuck putting up with me for the rest of our lives—Adrian, Maya, and Paloma (along with our fluffy menagerie, who are all critical in keeping the house functioning: snuggle-bunnies Chestnut, Apricot, and Buttercup, Luna the Floof, and the regal White Kitty). Anisa, none of this, or anything else I manage to do, would be possible without you.

About the Authors

IRVIN D. YALOM, MD, a visionary therapist and internationally bestselling author, is one of the world's foremost psychiatrists. He is the author of the *New York Times* bestseller *Love's Executioner*, *Momma and the Meaning of Life*, *When Nietzsche Wept*, *The Schopenhauer Cure*, and most recently *A Matter of Death and Life*, a dual memoir written with his late wife, Marilyn Yalom, PhD. His textbooks *The Theory and Practice of Group Psychotherapy* and *Existential Therapy* are standards for therapists in training worldwide. Dr. Yalom continues to live and write in Northern California.

BENJAMIN YALOM is a San Diego–based psychotherapist, creative coach, and longtime writing collaborator with his father, Irvin D. Yalom. Prior to his doctoral studies in marriage and family therapy, Benjamin was the visionary force behind foolsFURY theater, which helped transform San Francisco's performing arts scene in the early 2000s. He is also a graduate of the Iowa Writers' Workshop and an award-winning fiction writer.

www.yalomtherapy.com

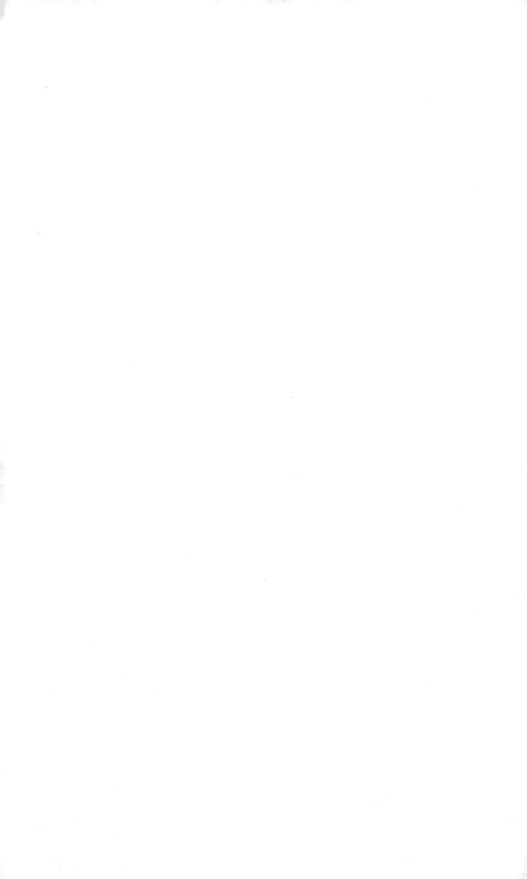